The
Endocrine
System

The
Endocrine
System

Titles in the Understanding the Human Body series include:

The Endocrine System

Pam Walker and Elaine Wood

LUCENT
BOOKS®

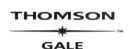

THOMSON

™

GALE

San Diego • Detroit • New York • San Francisco • Cleveland • New Haven, Conn. • Waterville, Maine • London • Munich

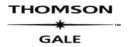

LIBRARY OF CONGRESS CATALOGING-IN-PUBLICATION DATA

Walker, Pam, 1958–
         The endocrine system / by Pam Walker and Elaine Wood.
      v. cm. — (Understanding the human body)
Includes bibliographical references and index.
Summary: Describes how the endocrine system works and the types of diseases and disorders.
         ISBN 1-59018-333-9 (hbk. : alk. paper)
   1. Endocrine glands—Juvenile literature. 2. Endocrinology—Juvenile literature.
[1. Endocrine glands.] I. Wood, Elaine, 1950– II. Title. III. Series.
         QP187 .W245 2003
         612.4—dc21

                                                                    2002015270

Printed in the United States of America

CONTENTS

FOREWORD

Since Earth first formed, countless creatures have come and gone. Dinosaurs and other types of land and sea animals fell prey to climatic shifts, food shortages, and myriad other environmental factors. Human beings survived throughout tens of thousands of years of evolution by adjusting to changes in climate and moving when food was scarce. The primary reason human beings were able to do this is that they possess a complex and adaptable brain and body.

The human body is comprised of organs, tissue, and bone that work independently and together to sustain life. Although it is both remarkable and unique, the human body shares features with other living organisms: the need to eat, breathe, and eliminate waste; the need to reproduce and eventually die.

Human beings, however, have many characteristics that other living creatures do not. The adaptable brain is responsible for these characteristics. Human beings, for example, have excellent memories; they can recall events that took place twenty, thirty, even fifty years earlier. Human beings also possess a high level of intelligence. Their unique capacity to invent, create, and innovate has led to discoveries and inventions such as vaccines, automobiles, and computers. And the human brain allows people to feel and respond to a variety of emotions. No other creature on Earth has such a broad range of abilities.

Although the human brain physically resembles a large, soft walnut, its capabilities seem limitless. The brain controls the body's movement, enabling humans to sprint, jog, walk, and crawl. It controls the body's internal functions, allowing people to breathe and maintain a heartbeat without effort. And it controls a person's creative talent, giving him or her the ability to write novels, paint masterpieces, or compose music.

Like a computer, the brain runs a network of body systems that keep human beings alive. The nervous system relays the brain's messages to the rest of the body. The respiratory system draws in life-sustaining oxygen and expels carbon dioxide waste. The circulatory system carries that oxygen to and from the body's vital organs. The reproductive system allows humans to continue their species and flourish as the dominant creatures on the planet. The digestive system takes in vital nutrients and converts them into the energy the body needs to grow. And the immune system protects the body from disease and foreign objects. When all of these systems work properly, the result is an intricate, extraordinary living machine.

Even when some of the systems are not working properly, the human body can often adapt. Healthy people have two kidneys, but, if necessary, they can live with just one. Doctors can remove a defective liver, heart, lung, or pancreas and replace it with a working one from another body. And a person blinded by an accident, disease, or birth defect can live a perfectly normal life by developing other senses to make up for the loss of sight.

The human body adapts to countless external factors as well. It sweats to cool off, adjusts the level of oxygen it needs at high altitudes, and derives nutritional value from a wide variety of foods, making do with what is available in a given region.

Only under tremendous duress does the human body cease to function. Extreme fluctuations in temperature, an invasion by hardy germs, or severe physical damage can halt normal bodily functions and cause death. Yet, even in such circumstances, the body continues to try to repair itself. The body of a diabetic, for example, will take in extra liquid and try to expel excess glucose through the urine. And a body exposed to extremely low temperatures will shiver in an effort to generate its own heat.

Lucent's Understanding the Human Body series explores different systems of the human body. Each volume describes the parts of a given body system and how they work both individually and collectively. Unique characteristics, malfunctions, and cutting edge medical procedures and technologies are also discussed. Photographs, diagrams, and glossaries enhance the text, and annotated bibliographies provide readers with opportunities for further discussion and research.

How the Endocrine System Works

Communication is the key to success in any organization, no matter how large or small. People communicate with one another in a variety of ways. A telephone call is a great way to carry on a conversation with one person; it is direct and personal. However, when people want to communicate with a group of individuals, the telephone may not be the most appropriate device. A more efficient way to reach a group is by broadcasting information by radio or television. Those who are interested tune in with a radio or television receiver. People who are not interested just ignore the information as it travels past them on invisible air waves.

The human body is an organization made of thousands of different tissues, each of which performs unique jobs to support the body as a whole. To work together, tissues must communicate and integrate their functions. To make a personal, direct contact, the nervous system carries a message from one tissue to another. The nervous system provides the shortest communication line, like the telephone. However, it cannot fill all of the communication needs because it is not equipped to broadcast signals to other large groups of cells. Broadcasting is the job of the endocrine system.

Broadcaster and Receiver

The endocrine system is made up of tissues that send messages and those that receive them. The specialized cells and tissues that create messages are endocrine glands. Glands are groups of tissue that produce and secrete a product. There are two different types of glands: endocrine and exocrine.

Endocrine glands discharge their goods either near the organ they control or into the body's blood system. The bloodstream is an intricate system of pathways that travels through the entire body, and it is a great tool for dispersing products. Exocrine glands release products onto some body surface through a tube or duct. The surface may be either internal or external. Sweat glands are good examples of exocrine glands. They make a liquid that flows through a sweat duct to the skin. Breasts are exocrine glands that discharge milk through ducts leading to the nipple.

The endocrine system relies on receivers called target organs to pick up the messages sent by glands.

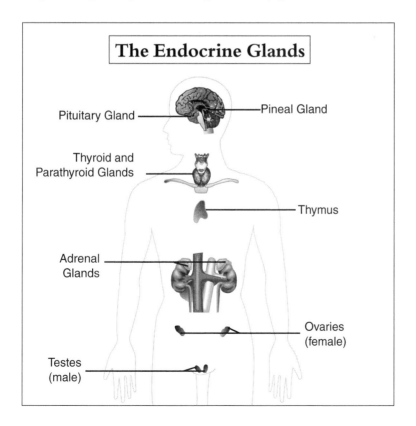

The Endocrine Glands

Pituitary Gland

Pineal Gland

Thyroid and Parathyroid Glands

Thymus

Adrenal Glands

Ovaries (female)

Testes (male)

Target organs are equipped with receptors on the surfaces of their cell membranes, like antennae on the roofs of houses, that pick up messages aimed at them. Target organs are the only tissues capable of receiving endocrine messages because other organs do not have the right kind of receptors or antennae. Endocrine messages affect target organs by changing the way, or the rate at which, they function.

The organs that make up the endocrine system are small and inconspicuous. Unlike body systems in which all of the organs are located together, or at least connected to one another, endocrine organs are scattered throughout the body. There are eleven individual endocrine glands, tucked away in the brain, neck, intestine, and body cavity. Even though they are small, their jobs are vital. Without these mass communication experts, the body could not function.

Some endocrine glands send out messages that are delivered to every cell in the body. For example, one gland transmits instructions on how to use glucose, the sugar that acts as cellular fuel. All cells depend on glucose for energy. Other endocrine glands put out messages that directly regulate only one or two body functions. Even so, their secretions have indirect effects on other body structures. One gland sends a message to the kidneys that determines how much water is removed from the body to make urine. However, the volume of water in the body indirectly affects levels of minerals in the blood as well as blood pressure.

The Messages

The endocrine system releases messages in the form of hormones. Hormones are chemicals produced in one part of the body that affect the activity of a specific group of cells and tissues within a target organ. Target organs may be adjacent to endocrine glands or located somewhere else in the body.

Knowledge about the structure and function of hormones is relatively recent. In the early 1900s, W. Bayliss and E. Starling accidentally found a hormone while studying the digestive system of dogs. They wanted to uncover the mechanism that triggers the release of digestive juices from the pancreas into the small intestine. They assumed that secretion of digestive juices was controlled by signals from the nervous system. To confirm their theory, they clipped the nerve supply to the upper intestine in experimental dogs. To their surprise, the dogs' pancreases continued to function. Equipped with the knowledge that the trigger was not a nerve impulse, they changed their theory and suggested that it might be a chemical. Eventually they were able to isolate the chemical and dubbed it secretin. Starling hypothesized that secretin was one of several chemicals that caused things to happen in the body. He coined the word *hormone*, from a Greek verb meaning "set into motion," to describe this group of chemicals.

Research over the last century has proved that Starling's term was fitting; all hormones literally arouse changes in target organs. The body produces many hormones, and individual ones affect organs in different ways. Some start chemical reactions while others cause processes to stop. Sometimes hormones speed up results, and at other times they slow them down. All in all, the body's hormones work together to maintain a stable internal environment.

Hormones are very powerful chemicals whose quantities must be precisely regulated. Too much or too little hormone can wreak havoc. Several mechanisms regulate hormone levels. In some cases, input from the nervous system determines how much hormone an endocrine gland will secrete. At other times, the concentration of some chemical in the blood triggers release of a hormone. Even the environment can switch one endocrine gland on or off. Yet the most common mechanism for regulating hormone levels is the negative feedback system.

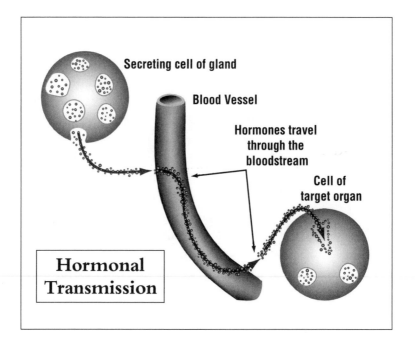

Secreting cell of gland

Blood Vessel

Hormones travel through the bloodstream

Cell of target organ

Hormonal Transmission

Stop and Go

In negative feedback, a system is turned off by the product it creates. After the product is released, the system receives constant updates about how much product is present. When levels of the product are high, the mechanism stops making it. When levels are low, the system starts again. A household thermostat is controlled by negative feedback. If the thermostat is set on 70 degrees F, its job is to maintain that temperature. When the air in the house is cooler than 70 degrees F, the thermostat signals the heating system to release its product, warm air. As warm air fills the house, the temperature steadily increases. When it reaches 70 degrees F, the thermostat signals the heating system to stop.

In the body, many endocrine glands are regulated by negative feedback. Such glands receive information from the hormones each one secretes. When the hormone reaches a certain level, this information, in the form of negative feedback, is what tells the endocrine gland to stop secreting. In a healthy body, this mechanism prevents the gland from producing too much hormone. As the body uses or consumes the hormone, its concentration goes down. In response to feedback indicating drops in hormone levels, the gland secretes hormone again. Negative feedback is a very effective system that keeps the blood levels of many hormones at a nearly constant level.

In Control: The Master Gland

Endocrine glands do not make and release hormones into the bloodstream all of the time. Individual glands have a boss that tells them when to work. They must be switched on by chemical signals from the pituitary gland, a grape-sized bump in the brain. Even though the pituitary is small, it is called the "master gland" because it controls the actions of several other endocrine glands. The area of the brain that holds the pituitary is the hypothalamus.

The hypothalamus serves two important roles in the endocrine system: it controls the pituitary and it makes

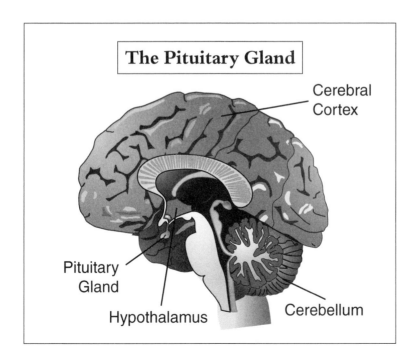

The Pituitary Gland

Cerebral Cortex

Pituitary Gland

Hypothalamus

Cerebellum

several hormones. In reality, the hypothalamus is the "master" of the "master gland" since one of its jobs is to regulate the activity of the pituitary. It does this by producing a specialized set of chemicals called releasing hormones. The pituitary does not have the power to act on its own; it must be exposed to releasing hormones before it can discharge it own hormones.

Storage Chamber → *a posterior pituitary*

The pituitary gland has two distinct jobs, each conducted in a different area of the gland: anterior and posterior. The posterior, or rear, portion of the pituitary gland does not contain cells that make hormones. Instead, it serves as a storage chamber that holds antidiuretic hormone (ADH) and oxytocin (OT), two chemicals made by nerve cells in the hypothalamus, which drain into the posterior part of the gland. The secretion of these two hormones is not controlled by releasing hormones, however; they enter the bloodstream only when signaled to do so by the nervous system.

An antidiuretic is a substance that decreases urine production, and thus a person's two kidneys are the target organs of ADH. As an antidiuretic, ADH helps maintain water in the body by reducing the amount of water that kidneys excrete. If a person's body is low on water, or dehydrated, the posterior lobe releases ADH, which travels via blood to the kidneys. As a result, less water is used to produce urine. However, if the body has excess water, the release of ADH is inhibited, allowing the kidneys to produce urine and keep the body's water levels normal.

Oxytocin also has some antidiuretic qualities, but not as many as ADH. In women and other female mammals, the primary target organs of oxytocin are the uterus and breasts. During childbirth, this hormone causes contractions of the muscles in the uterus. After childbirth, it stimulates the contraction of cells in milk-producing ducts of the breasts, forcing milk to the nipples. Nursing baby animals, such as kittens or puppies, demonstrates one of the mechanisms that release oxytocin. As they suckle, they knead their mothers' mammary glands with their feet. This kneading stimulates nerve endings that send signals to the brain to discharge milk. As a result, oxytocin is released, which in turn causes the release of milk.

Production Department → *Anterior pituitary*

The anterior, or forward, part of the pituitary is made up of several different types of glandular tissue, each of which makes a different product. As a result, this gland generates six different hormones. Four of the hormones are classified as trophic hormones because their job is to control the activity of other endocrine glands. The trophic hormones are thyroid-stimulating hormone (TSH),

Puppies work furiously to obtain milk from their mother by kneading her mammary glands.

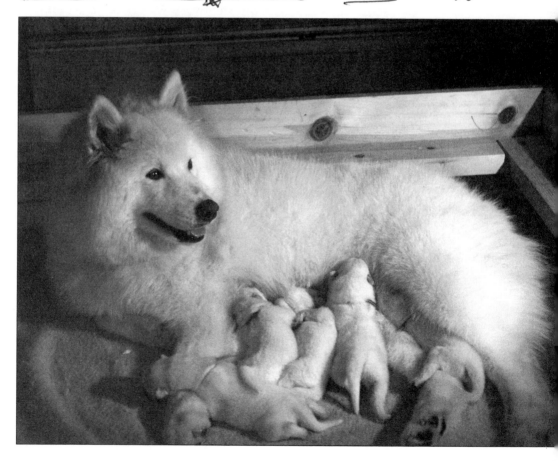

adrenocorticotropic hormone (ACTH), follicle-stimulating hormone (FSH), and luteinizing hormone (LH). The other two hormones made in the anterior pituitary are prolactin and growth hormone (GH).

As its name implies, TSH regulates secretion of hormones produced by the thyroid gland. ACTH controls the production of hormones by the adrenal cortex, the outer layer of the adrenal gland. FSH and LH, known collectively as gonadotropins, or gonad growers, regulate gonads, or sexual organs. In females, FSH acts on the ovaries, the organs that produce eggs. It stimulates ovaries to complete two tasks: mature some of the egg cells contained within them and make female sex hormones. When an egg cell has reached maturity, LH triggers its release from the ovary. Women are also influenced by the hormone prolactin, which causes milk production after the birth of a baby. In males, FSH works in concert with LH to regulate production of sperm, male reproductive cells, and testosterone, the male sex hor-

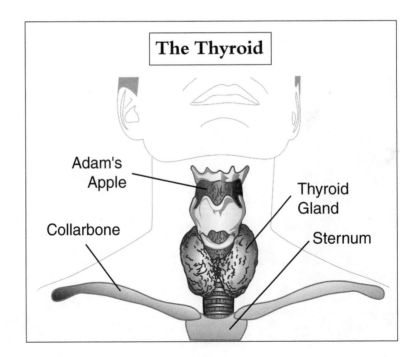

The Thyroid

Adam's Apple

Thyroid Gland

Collarbone

Sternum

mone. The role of prolactin in males is not well understood.

Growth hormone is classified as a general metabolic hormone because it affects the way cells work throughout the body. GH stimulates body cells to grow and divide. It also helps new cells take up and use nutrients. Much of its effort is directed at the growth of long bones and at the muscles that attach to bones. Therefore, GH has an influence on mature body size.

The Vital Thyroid

Release of TSH by the anterior pituitary activates the thyroid gland, TSH's target organ. The thyroid is located in the front of the neck, directly below the Adam's apple. Made of two sections, or lobes, connected by a thin strip of tissue, the thyroid has a butterfly shape. The secreting cells in the thyroid produce three hormones: thyroxine, triiodothyronine, and calcitonin.

Thyroxine and triiodothyronine have similar jobs, although triiodothyronine is three to four times stronger than its cousin. These two chemicals help regulate the rate at which glucose is used by cells to make energy. Since all cells must produce energy to power their activities, these thyroid hormones are vital to a person's survival. To produce these two hormones, the thyroid must be supplied with iodine, an element usually present in the diet.

Like other hormones, calcitonin is involved in regulation. However, it does not regulate glucose levels. Calcitonin helps control the amount of calcium and phosphate in the blood. Calcium and phosphate have essential functions in several organ systems, so these minerals must be carefully distributed. They play roles in balancing water and mineral levels in blood, conducting messages along nerves, contracting muscles, clotting blood, and building bones and teeth. If there is an excess of calcium in the blood, the anterior pituitary releases calcitonin. As a result, calcium in the bloodstream is absorbed into bone, and both calcium and phosphorus are excreted by the kidneys, thereby lowering the levels of these minerals in the blood.

Four parathyroid glands are located on the back of the thyroid. Even though they are close together, the thyroid and parathyroid glands do not function in the same manner. Each parathyroid is a small, yellow-brown mass of hormone-secreting cells that are surrounded and supplied by millions of tiny blood vessels. Parathyroid hormone (PTH) works with calcitonin to regulate calcium levels in the blood. These two hormones have an antagonistic relationship: The effect of one opposes the effect of the other. Whereas calcitonin reduces levels of calcium in the blood, PTH, activated when calcium levels in the blood drop, increases blood calcium. The target organs for this hormone are bones, kidneys, and the small intestine. Bone releases stored calcium into the bloodstream when signaled to do so by PTH. PTH also raises calcium levels by causing the kidneys to retain calcium. In the small intestine, PTH increases absorption of calcium from food, raising blood levels even more. Levels of PTH are controlled by negative feedback. When calcium concentration is low, PTH is secreted; however, when blood levels of calcium increase, PTH is inhibited.

Dual-Functioning Adrenal Glands

A bean-shaped adrenal gland sits on top of each human kidney. The name *adrenal* is derived from the Latin prefix *ad*, meaning "near," and the word *renal*, referring to the kidneys. Each gland functions like two distinct endocrine organs. The central portion of an adrenal gland is called the medulla, and the outer layer is referred to as the cortex.

Cells of the medulla, deep within each adrenal gland, are interwoven with small blood vessels and nerve cells. Medulla cells secrete two similar hormones: epinephrine (also called adrenaline) and norepinephrine, or noradrenaline. These chemicals have amazingly similar structures

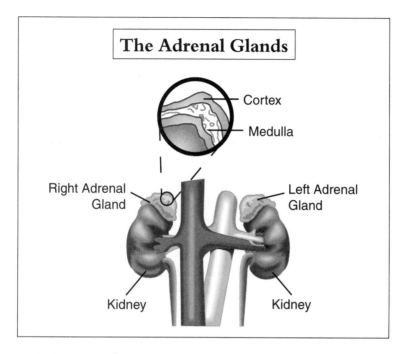

The Adrenal Glands

Cortex

Medulla

Right Adrenal Gland

Left Adrenal Gland

Kidney

Kidney

and functions. In fact, most epinephrine is made from norepinephrine.

When the body is under stress, nerve fibers stimulate the adrenal medullas, causing them to pump their hormones into the bloodstream. Epinephrine and norepinephrine increase the heart rate, strengthen the heartbeat, elevate blood pressure, speed up breathing, and slow digestive processes. Together, these changes get more oxygen and glucose into the blood and raise thinking to a higher level of alertness. In this way they prepare the body to deal with danger.

The outermost layer of each adrenal gland is referred to as the cortex, which produces aldosterone, cortisol, and sex hormones. Aldosterone is a hormone that helps regulate the amount of water and minerals, or electrolytes, in the body. It does so by directing the kidneys either to remove minerals from the blood or to leave the minerals in the kidneys to be flushed out of the body in urine. Sodium is one of the important minerals controlled by this hormone. When aldosterone levels are high, kidneys reabsorb sodium traveling through them and return it to the bloodstream. When sodium is reabsorbed, so is water. Therefore, aldosterone also affects blood volume, or the amount of water in the blood. As the blood volume increases, so does blood pressure. Consequently, aldosterone indirectly influences blood pressure.

Cortisol, another adrenal cortex hormone, has the job of keeping blood glucose levels constant. Since glucose fuels cells, cortisol targets every cell in the body. When advised by negative feedback that glucose levels are low, this hormone conserves glucose in several ways. It slows the assembly of proteins from their building blocks, leaving these materials (amino acids) in the blood so they can be used as fuel in place of glucose. It promotes the use of fat as a source of energy, again reducing the use of glucose. Cortisol causes cells in the liver to make glucose from other nutrients, increasing levels of glucose in the blood.

Cortisol also affects wound healing. Its presence slows swelling after an injury and helps reduce discomfort by inhibiting the release of pain-causing secretions called prostaglandins. This is why cortisol-like drugs are often prescribed as medications for patients with conditions that cause pain and swelling, such as arthritis and asthma.

In both sexes, the adrenals produce fairly small amounts of male hormones of the type called adrenal androgens. Androgens in females are converted to estrogen, the female hormone. Since most of the sex hormones in both males and females are made by reproductive tissues, the roles of adrenal sex hormones are not clear. They may simply act as supplementary supplies, augmenting the primary reproductive glands. Some research indicates that they affect the female sex drive.

Creating the Next Generation

In females, the reproductive glands, or gonads, are the ovaries, almond-shaped organs in the pelvic cavity. Ovaries produce female sex cells, called eggs, or ova, and

two female hormones, estrogen and progesterone.
Estrogen has several jobs. It stimulates the maturation of
reproductive organs and the development of secondary
sex characteristics (such as widening of the hips, the
development of breasts, and the appearance of pubic
hair).

Estrogen also helps maintain pregnancy and prepare
breasts to produce milk. Working with progesterone,
estrogen prepares the uterus to receive a fertilized egg.

The gonads of males are testes, paired organs suspend-
ed outside the body in a sac called the scrotum. Testes
manufacture male sex cells, sperm, and the male hormone testosterone. Testosterone brings about the development of secondary sex characteristics (such as the
growth of facial hair, broadening of the shoulders, and
lowering of the voice), maturation of the reproductive
system, and development of the male sex drive.

Crucial Cells in the Pancreas

The pancreas is a long organ located in the body cavity
behind the stomach. The pancreas is actually two organs
rolled into one; it is made up of tissues for both an
endocrine and an exocrine gland. The exocrine part of
the pancreas makes digestive juices that flow through a
duct to the upper end of the small intestine. The
endocrine portion is made up of thousands of small
patches of cells scattered through the pancreas. Called
islets of Langerhans, these patches contain two types of
cells: alpha and beta.

Both work to maintain stable levels of glucose in the
blood, but in opposite ways. Alpha cells produce the hormone called glucagon, and beta cells make another hormone, insulin.

Several hours after a meal or after periods of exercise,
glucose levels in the blood are low. If glucose drops
extremely low, cells in the body cannot make energy,
and loss of consciousness or death can occur. Before the
situation becomes dangerous, moderately low levels of

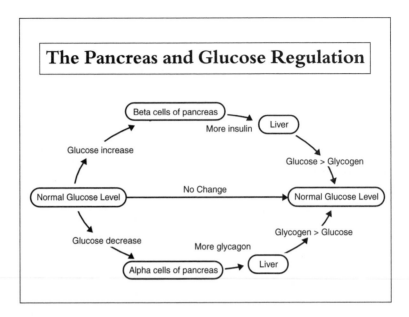

The Pancreas and Glucose Regulation

glucose trigger the release of glucagon from alpha cells. This hormone stimulates the liver to change glycogen, a stored form of glucose, into glucose, thus raising blood levels of this life-sustaining sugar. In healthy people, this negative feedback mechanism ensures that the blood will never be so low in glucose that cells cannot function.

The effect of insulin is the opposite of that of glucagon; it lowers the blood levels of glucose. Also regulated by negative feedback, insulin is released after a meal when glucose is abundant in the body. Insulin enables glucose to diffuse through the cell membranes, making it possible for the molecule to move from the blood into the cells. Insulin also acts on the liver to stimulate the formation of glycogen from glucose, further lowering blood levels.

Since the norm for human beings is to sleep at night and eat during the day, glucagon is primarily secreted during the night and insulin during the day. Daily fluctuations in these hormone levels are a function of personal eating habits. However, secretions of another gland, the pineal, are not affected by one's activities. The pineal is in charge of telling the body when to rest and when to play.

Hidden Hormone Sources

Hormones are produced in small patches of tissue in several other areas of the body: the brain, intestine, kidneys, placenta, and thymus gland. The pineal gland in the brain is unique among endocrine glands because it is stimulated by a cue from the environment, light. This gland has undergone some evolutionary changes over time. Until about 240 million years ago, all of the animals with backbones possessed a light-sensitive organ, which was located on top of the head. This eye triggered the pineal gland. A modified form of this ancient, or a type of "third eye," organ still exists in the brain.

The pineal gland is a petite structure located deep within the brain tissue. Its job is to secrete melatonin. The amount of this hormone released by the pineal depends on the amount of light in the environment. Since light does not shine directly on the pineal gland, this organ gets information about light from the nerves that connect the eyes to the brain. When it is dark, nerve impulses from the eyes travel at a lower frequency than they do when it is light. The low-frequency transmissions trigger increased production of melatonin by the pineal gland. Melatonin targets certain cells in the brain that help regulate sleep behavior. When melatonin levels are high, these nerve cells are activated, and they prepare the body for sleep. When the sun comes up in the morning, melatonin production drops, and the body wakes up.

The Glands Rule

The organs that are classified together as the endocrine system are spread throughout the body. They work with the nervous system to transmit messages to cells and to integrate and control the body's functions. In this way, endocrine glands help keep the chemical environment of cells fairly constant.

Endocrine glands do not have a free hand; they operate under many restraints. The "master gland," or pituitary, produces hormones that dominate other endocrine glands, including the thyroid, adrenal cortex, ovaries, and testes. The pituitary, in turn, is ruled by the true power behind the throne, the hypothalamus. The hypothalamus is part of the nervous system, where it supervises internal organs and acts in response to emotions.

Many of the endocrine glands work together to regulate the same function. Some, like insulin and glucagon, have an antagonistic relationship in which one raises levels of a chemical while the other lowers levels. This tug-of-war mechanism keeps the chemical at optimal levels in the blood. Others require the sum total of two or more hormones to produce the desired effect on the target organ. For example, prolactin, oxytocin, estrogen, and progesterone are all necessary for the production of milk in breasts. A few hormones can only exert their effects after other hormones have primed the target organ. Pregnancy can only occur if estrogen prepares the uterus for the effects of progesterone. Working as a team, these glands control thousands of chemical reactions that are essential to the survival of a human being.

2 Life with Stress

All living things share the instinct of self-preservation. After all, the goal in life is to live long enough to reproduce and propagate the species. Along with the will to survive, animals are equipped with physiological systems and natural behaviors that help make that goal a true possibility. The endocrine system provides some of the most important tools in the survival toolbox.

When faced with physical danger, a human or any other animal has one of two choices: take a stand and fight or make a run for safety. In either the "fight" or the "flight" scenario, the body must be primed and ready for action. It is the job of the endocrine system to gather glucose to provide the muscles with energy and to heighten senses and reflexes so that the body can perform at its best.

Survival has not always been a simple task. The lives of early humans were very difficult. They hunted animals for food while protecting themselves from predators that viewed them as meals. Some groups of humans moved often in search of water, better hunting grounds, or new sources of plant food, and they were threatened by other groups of people in disputes over territory or resources. Danger was part of everyday life. For these people, it was literally true that the strongest survived.

Only in the last few decades have scientists explored the complex physical changes that occur in the body of a person confronted with danger. Research that began in the early

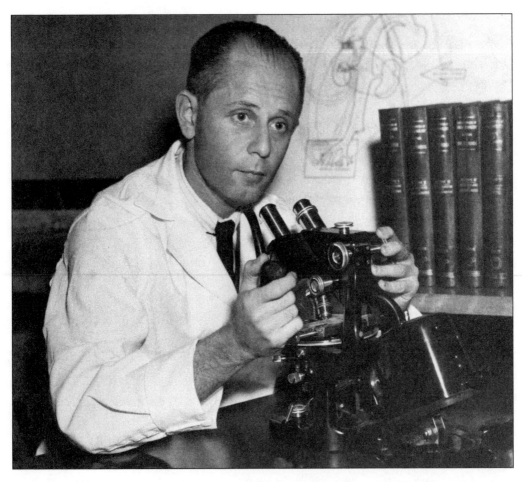

Hans Seyle discovered and named stress. His pioneering paper explained how stress changes the body and affects health.

1900s is ongoing in an effort to learn more about the body's tactics for staying alive under desperate conditions. The scientist who first detected some of these strategies did so by accident.

Early Research

In 1935, Hans Selye, a research scientist at McGill University in Montreal, was conducting experiments to learn more about sex hormones. His goal was to find out if the body secreted sex hormones in addition to estrogen, progesterone, and testosterone, the chemicals already known to affect sexual development. He designed an experiment to find out. He injected several groups of rats with different combinations of extracts from two structures: ovaries and placenta. Ovaries are the female reproductive organs that make eggs, and the placenta is a sac that surrounds a fetus as it develops inside of its mother. If another sex hormone existed, he expected the rats' bodies to produce it in response to some or all of his injections.

However, Selye's experiments did not yield the expected results. He had thought that different injections would stimulate the rats' bodies in different ways. Yet, he found that no matter what combination of extracts he gave a group of rats, all of the animals responded in the same manner. In every case, the rats' bodies underwent three distinct changes: One of their endocrine organs enlarged, organs of their defense system shriveled, and bleeding sores developed in their stomachs.

Not knowing how to interpret these results, Selye decided to continue his experiment. He injected a variety of materials into the rats, including extracts from other organs as well as chemicals, still trying to provoke different changes in their bodies. He found that no matter what substances he injected into the rats, they experienced the same three changes.

Selye finally concluded that he had discovered a new syndrome, or set of symptoms that occurs together in response to a disease. However, he did not know to what disease the rats were responding. In his experiments, the animals seemed to be reacting to a host of different problems. No matter what injurious agents he injected into them, the rats all showed the same response.

After rethinking his experiments, Selye decided that the rats did have one thing in common: They were all receiving an unnatural stimulus. Therefore, their responses did fit the definition of a "syndrome." Selye dubbed the new syndrome "stress," and he used the word "stressors" to describe the agents that produced stress. He also coined the term "general adaptation syndrome" to describe the physical changes that occurred in the rats' bodies in response to the stressors. In 1956, he presented his classic paper, "The Stress of Life," in which he explained how stress itself changes the body, producing problems and symptoms that had been misunderstood for years. His pioneering work in the field of stress gave the medical community new insights into the way life situations can affect health.

Current Ideas

Today, scientists have used Selye's research as a platform from which to expand and refine the world's understanding of stress. The definition of "stressor" has been broadened to include any agent or stimulus that produces stress. Since a stimulus is anything that provokes a physical response, noise, a thorn, a feather, or even a scary situation can qualify as a stressor. Stressors are often extreme stimuli, too much or too little of something. For example, very hot or very cold conditions stress the body; moderate environments rarely cause problems for people. Extremely loud noises can be stressors, but so can total silence. Too much food can be a stressor, as can too little food.

Overcrowded living conditions, where there is excessive contact with others, is stressful; so is total isolation. In general, any injurious or painful stimulus causes stress on the body. An illness, such as a case of the flu, causes stress-related changes in the body. So does an injury like a broken leg or a sprained wrist.

Real dangers are not the only stressors; they can also include conditions that a person wrongly perceives as dangerous. For most people, being in a truly dangerous situation arouses fear and anxiety, setting off stress changes in the body. If an assailant holds a victim at gunpoint, the victim's body shows signs of stress. Yet, a person who fears escalators might experience the same kind of stress reaction riding escalators in a department store, and one who is afraid of speaking in public can undergo a similar response when walking out on the stage. Even the thought of danger or an experience such as a scary movie or wild roller coaster can set off the stress response.

Stress can be very personal. The events that cause stress in one person may not elicit the same reaction from someone else. Loud noises might be extremely stressful to one individual, but not to another. Not only do stressors differ greatly from one person to the next; they can even vary from day to day in the same person. Heavy traffic may be a stressor on Monday morning, but not on Tuesday. The condition of one's mind, the events in life, the amount of rest one has had, as well as many other factors affect whether or not events act as stressors.

Everyone reacts differently to stress. Heavy traffic can challenge one person and terrify another.

Despite all this variety, all stressors, no matter what their origin, have the same effect on the body. Just as Seyle's rats

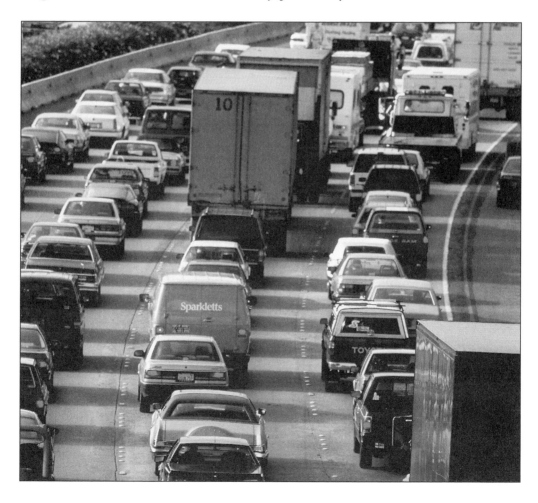

experienced three physical changes, people undergo some common changes when exposed to stress. This is because all stress acts on the hypothalamus in two ways. First, it directly stimulates the hypothalamus, causing it to secrete hormones. One of these is a releasing hormone called corticotrophin-releasing hormone (CRH). At the same time, another hypothalamic hormone stimulates one of the nerve centers of the brain, as well as two other important endocrine glands. Second, stressors affect the emotional part of the brain, an area called the limbic lobe. This emotional center works directly with the hypothalamus, providing it with information. All of these changes in the brain and endocrine glands produce the physical transformations called the "stress syndrome" or "stress response."

Stress Syndrome

Once a stressor has set off the hypothalamus and the limbic lobe, a predictable cascade of events begins. Stimulation of the hypothalamus releases cortisol and ACTH into the bloodstream. Cortisol's job is to make glucose available to the muscles. ACTH from the adrenal medulla reduces urine output.

At the same time, the brain sends a signal to the adrenal medulla that something is wrong, prodding it to dump lots of adrenaline into the bloodstream. Adrenaline starts the series of reactions known collectively as the "fight or flight" response. Immediately, heart rate and respiration increase, blood pressure shoots up, blood glucose levels rise, and the pupils dilate. Next, endorphins, natural pain killers, are released to provide instant relief from any pain that may result as a consequence of the stressful situation. Secretions slow, so the mouth produces very little saliva and becomes dry. At the same time, the hands and the soles of the feet feel sweaty, and the body color pales. The body makes the most of its resources by prioritizing, sending extra blood to muscles and the brain, but taking blood away from the digestive system, kidneys, liver, and areas of the brain that are not critical in a combat situation, like the region controlling speech.

All of these changes are designed to get the body primed and ready to deal with a threat. With highly oxygenated blood pounding through vessels, glucose pouring into the blood for fuel, senses heightened, and pain-deadening chemicals in circulation, the body is ready to take care of any danger that presents itself.

Stress Hormones in Action

Much of the body's response to stress depends on the work of two hormones: adrenaline and cortisol. Adrenaline puts the body in a state of excitement so it can cope with the challenge. Cortisol mobilizes energy stores so the muscles can respond to the stressor.

Cortisol is a complex hormone, and it has both short- and long-term effects. In the short run, cortisol gets glucose to muscles to enhance their activity. It also suppresses the immune response so that if an injury occurs during the dangerous situation, swelling and pain that would interfere with the body's ability to fight or flee will be minimized.

If the danger or stressor is not resolved in a few hours, cortisol remains in the bloodstream for an extended period, and suppression of the immune system continues. This can have negative consequences because swelling is a normal part of healing and repair, and without this mechanism healing is hampered. Inactivation of the immune system for long periods of time causes a reduction in the number of disease-fighting cells that are present in the body. Consequently, cortisol makes the body more prone to infection. In its glucose-supplying role, cortisol eventually takes on a new job: It tries to restore the supplies of glucose that may have been used up during the emergency situation. Therefore, cortisol in the system encourages food intake to prepare the body for an extended crisis.

Adrenaline, the hormone that creates fear and excitement, reduces fatigue and gives the body a "rush," or feeling of energy. Once released from the adrenal medulla, adrenaline reaches its target organs in a matter of seconds. Its presence is responsible for increasing blood flow and heart

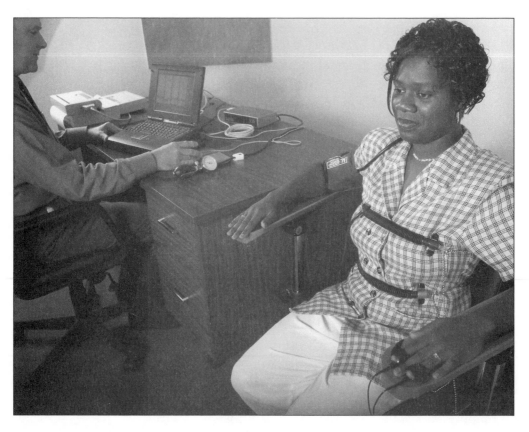

A woman takes a polygraph test. The test measures physical reactions as a person answers questions.

rate, rerouting blood to the extremities, dilating the pupils, and focusing the pupils for keener distance vision.

Physical and Psychological Stresses

Stressors can come from many sources, both physical and psychological. Physical stress results from conditions imposed on the body, whereas psychological stress is caused by conditions occurring in the mind. However, conditions of these two types often overlap and are difficult to separate. Physical stress can lead to psychological stress, and the reverse is true. Psychological stress may produce some emotional responses, such as anxiety, depression, or guilt. However, it also leads to physical symptoms, such as a rush of energy or a depressed immune system, or behavioral changes like fidgeting, quarreling, lying, or crying. The close relationship of psychological and physical stress gives some insight into the powerful link between feelings, thoughts, and the body.

The ancient Chinese knew that stress, whether of physical or psychological origin, could cause physical changes. A person suspected of lying was made to chew rice powder and then spit it out. If the powder was not moistened by saliva, the interrogators knew they had not been told the truth. Psychological stress, like that caused by deception, dries up saliva. Today, the same logic is used in an investigative tool called the polygraph machine. Polygraph tests, often improperly called lie detector tests, are designed to monitor the body's responses in a stressful situation. The stress caused by lying creates measurable physical changes in the bodies of most people.

In a polygraph test, the subject sits in a chair, and several tubes and wires are wrapped around the body at specific locations. Two rubber tubes are placed around the subject's chest to measure the rate of respiration. A cuff is wrapped around the upper arm to monitor changes in blood pressure. Small plates that measure the amount of sweat produced are attached to the fingers. As the examiner asks a series of questions, the subject answers, and physiological changes are recorded. Since some individuals do not experience stress when they are lying and others find it stressful simply to be under suspicion and subjected to a polygraph examination, the so-called lie detector does not detect lies; it does, however, detect changes that occur in the body and may or may not indicate accurately that a lie has been told.

Stages of Adrenaline Action

Not all of the changes caused by the release of adrenaline happen at one time; they occur in stages. The emergency or alarm response is Stage One. When danger is perceived, the adrenal medulla dumps adrenaline into the bloodstream, increasing heart rate and respiration. One feels super-alert, powerful, and ready to take on anything. During Stage One the problem may be resolved. If so, the stress response will end.

If the problem persists, the body moves to the next stage. By the time Stage Two arrives, the body has stopped pouring adrenaline into the blood but continues to release it in a small, steady stream to keep the body on alert. Very quickly adrenaline uses up all the body's stores of energy. In this stage, a person feels driven or pressured. In a short time, fatigue sets in, but the anxiety produced by adrenaline makes it difficult to rest. If the stressor is finally eliminated, the stress response ends.

However, some stressors cannot be removed from life quickly or easily. They continue, day in and day out, for weeks, months, or years. In this case, the body enters Stage Three. In this condition, the body's need for energy is greater than its ability to produce energy. A person who has become chronically stressed develops symptoms such as insomnia, personality changes, depression, and fatigue. In extreme cases, death can result.

Today's World with Yesterday's Body

Today humans live in a genetically identical copy of the body that belonged to their ancestors, a body with an efficient endocrine response for surviving dangerous situations. However, people today rarely find themselves facing the threats of wild animals or belligerent neighboring tribes, situations where "fight or flight" is an appropriate response.

Modern-day stressors exist, but they are different from the ones that plagued prehistoric people. Stress comes from a variety of sources. It may be related to issues at school: too much homework, critical teachers, or rude students. Stressors in the workplace, such as disorganization and unrealistic expectations, are common. Home can even be a source of stress, where lack of family support or ineffective parenting causes problems.

These stressors evoke the same responses in modern man that an attack by wild animals induced in people millions of years ago. If a parent reprimands an adolescent son about poor grades in school, the youth's body goes into Stage

One, and adrenaline pours into his blood. As a result, heart rate, blood pressure, and respiration increase. Yet, this stressor cannot be eliminated with a fight or by running to a safer location. It has to be dealt with in a different way. If the stress is ignored, it can progress to Stage Two or even to Stage Three.

To resolve stress, one must first recognize it. The wild feelings that result from stress can often be brought under control. One way to slow or stop a strong surge of adrenaline is to engage in an activity that uses a lot of muscle, such as exercise, so that the adrenaline can be used up. Once the adrenaline chain reaction is broken, the body will usually return to its normal, nonstressed state.

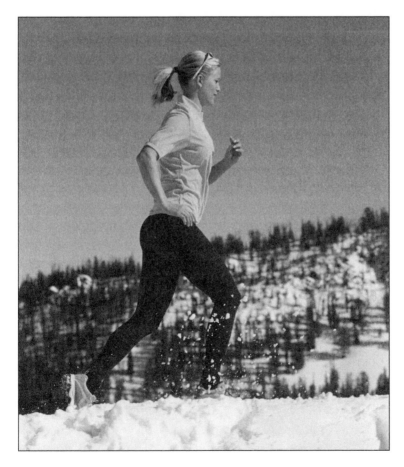

Vigorous physical exercise releases stress by using muscles the body has prepared for the "fight or flight" reaction.

The Effects of Stress

Selye used the term "general adaptation syndrome" to explain a set of responses that he believed enabled the body to adapt to, or deal with, a stressful situation. Yet he also knew that not all stressful stimuli or situations can be successfully resolved. He suggested that when resolution is not possible, the body will adapt, but the adaptation will be to develop a disease. In a series of experiments, he exposed animals to intensely stressful stimuli. As he expected, the animals developed unhealthy conditions, including high blood pressure, arthritis, and arteriosclerosis.

Today scientists have demonstrated that stress has both negative and positive effects. Some stress helps motivate people to finish a task, beat the clock, or conquer a problem. However, long-term stress can be dangerous. High levels of cortisol in the blood for extended periods of time curb the immune system, so it becomes more difficult to recover from illness. Stress also raises blood pressure and speeds the rate at which fatty materials are deposited on the inside of blood vessels, increasing the risk of heart attack and stroke. Stress has an impact on mental health as well. It decreases the ability to think through problems and explain ideas, leading to confusion. Depression has also been shown to be related to stress.

A pregnant woman's stress can affect the health of her unborn child. This is partly due to the fact that when a woman is very anxious, blood flow to the uterus is reduced. Since uterine arteries supply food and oxygen to the developing fetus, stress can restrict the amount of nutrients a baby receives. Additionally, high levels of cortisol in the mother can cross the sac that holds the baby and increase levels of cortisol in the baby's blood. The development of the baby's brain is sensitive to cortisol, just as it is sensitive to alcohol, tobacco, and other drugs.

The Sum of Stress

The body undergoes several normal changes when subjected to stress. In the past, these changes helped humans

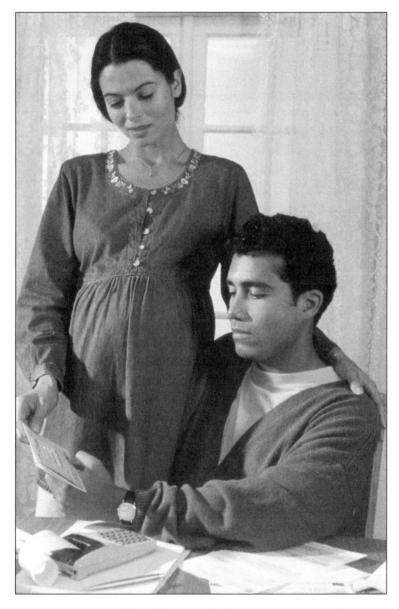

survive by providing them with the energy needed to stay alive in a dangerous situation. If a person encountered a lion, quick escape was imperative. To run, the body needed plenty of energy and oxygen for the muscles. The bodies of early humans geared up for danger by dumping stress hormones into the bloodstream. Two hormones, cortisol and adrenaline, were instrumental in preparing the body.

Humans in the twenty-first century live out their lives in bodies genetically indistinguishable from those of their remote ancestors. Now, however, the environment has greatly changed. In the developed world, danger rarely lurks around the corner, and the stress reactions that served early man so well are not as useful to his modern counterpart. In fact, some of the body's programmed responses to stress may actually cause illness.

Stress can have negative or positive effects on the body. Positive stress, called eustress, helps motivate people to accomplish tasks and solve problems. But negative stress, distress, can be a danger when it lingers for long periods, possibly leading to both physical and mental disorders.

3 | Puberty and Adolescence

Animals are not born in their adult form. When animals first appear in the world, they are often very different from their parents. The youngsters of frogs, land-dwelling, air-breathing amphibians, are nothing like the adults they will become. Baby frogs emerge from soft, gelatinous eggs as small, legless creatures equipped with gills and tails for living in water. Gradually, they mature into four-legged terrestrials like their parents.

Many insects go through even more astonishing changes in their journeys from birth to adulthood. Butterflies are not born with wings and delicate antennae. Instead they hatch as small worm-shaped larvae that are designed for eating and growing. Eventually, these larvae wrap themselves in a cocoon of their own making in which their bodies take on the sexually mature adult configurations.

The offspring of mammals more closely resemble the adults than do the babies of frogs, butterflies, and countless other creatures. Mammals are animals that are covered with hair and feed their young on milk from mammary glands. However, young mammals are small and weak, so, like other animals, they must go through several important stages of growth and development.

Human young spend more time growing and maturing than do the babies of any other mammals. At birth, a human is completely dependent on its parents for food and

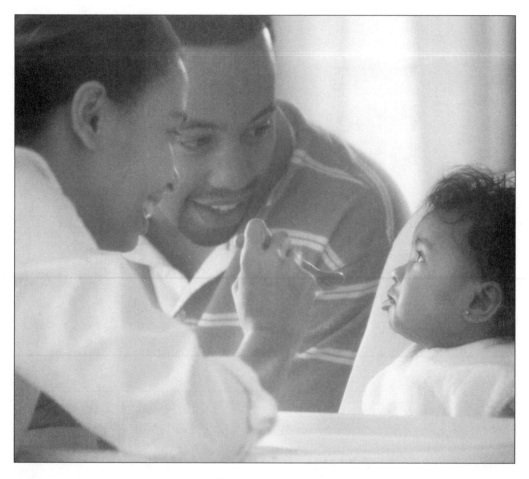

Human babies learn and grow rapidly when caring adults provide food and care.

care. A well-nourished baby grows at a rapid rate, often increasing in body length by 50 percent during each of the first three years of life. By age three, a young human's growth slows somewhat. During this stage of life, called childhood, humans grow about two or three inches a year. Children are able to do many things for themselves but are still very dependent on parents and family relationships. The last stage of growth for humans is puberty, which begins at about nine years of age. The term "puberty" refers to the dramatic physical changes in the human body that culminate in sexual maturation. At the end of this time of growth and change, a young person is a sexually mature being, capable of propagating the species.

The Time of Change

"Puberty" and "adolescence" are two terms that are sometimes used interchangeably. However, they do not mean exactly the same thing. Puberty is a portion of adolescence, the part concerning physical, hormonal, and sexual changes. Adolescence includes all the changes between childhood and adulthood—social and psychological, as well as physical. It is an important period of development during which a young person learns how to be an adult.

The changes associated with maturation in all animals, from insects to humans, are controlled by hormones. Growth and development are complex procedures, involving more than just an increase in the number of cells; these events also change the way cells function. Therefore, transformations of the body must be highly orchestrated so that the end result is an organism that is physically and psychologically ready for the jobs of adulthood.

The mechanisms that start puberty are not completely understood, but scientists do know that hormones play a major role. During childhood, the brain actually inhibits puberty by setting the body's hormones on low. About the time of puberty, rising levels of androgens signal the brain to remove some of its restrictions, and more hormones are released.

At a certain age, the hypothalamus, the part of the brain that controls most endocrine functions, sends out gonadotropin-releasing hormone, GnRH. When GnRH reaches the pituitary, it stimulates this gland to send out three products: growth hormone, LH, and FSH. In boys, these LH and FSH hormones trigger the production of testosterone and sperm. In girls, they stimulate the ovaries to make estrogen and start forming mature eggs. In both sexes, growth hormone is responsible for the tremendous increase in size.

Shared Experiences

Puberty generally begins between ages nine and sixteen, depending on factors such as heredity, nutrition, stress, general health, and gender. Release of hormones causes a multitude of alterations in both males and females. Some of these changes are specific to sex, but others occur in boys and girls alike. One of the surest hallmarks of puberty is an increase in height and weight. Young people experience a dramatic growth spurt. Girls begin this spurt at a younger age than do boys. During puberty, young people may grow a total of twelve inches in height and gain twenty to thirty pounds.

Both sexes gain fat, although girls gain more than boys. By the end of puberty, boys are usually more muscular and stronger than females. The average muscle-to-fat ratio of boys is 3 to 1; in girls it is 5 to 4. Therefore, boys are physically stronger than girls. They also have larger hearts and lungs relative to body size. Boys have a lower resting heart rate because their larger heart muscle can pump more blood around the body with every beat. The blood of boys has greater oxygen-carrying ability, more hemoglobin—the molecule that carries oxygen in red blood cells—and more red blood cells than the blood of girls. As a general rule, by the end of puberty boys possess a greater capacity for strength and endurance than girls.

Most boys and girls develop acne in adolescence. No one knows exactly why, although it is well documented that fluctuations in hormone levels trigger eruptions on the skin. That is why acne may also accompany a menstrual cycle, pregnancy, menopause, or the use of hormone supplements like birth control pills. Acne in young people is primarily thought to be due to increases in levels of androgens. The low levels of androgens in childhood explain why acne rarely appears before puberty.

Acne begins in the skin's sebaceous glands, which secrete an oily substance called sebum into hair follicles. Sebum's job is to lubricate hairs. Normally, this thick liquid flows out of hair follicles through pores to the surface of the skin. Production of sebum increases sharply during puberty. This excess sebum, combined with bacteria that normally live within hair follicles, can form a plug called a comedo that

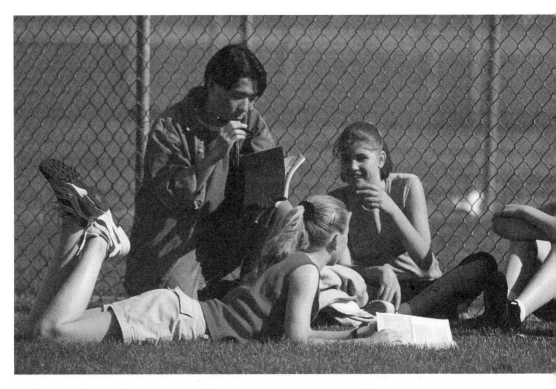

stops up the follicle. If a follicle is blocked at the surface of skin, the plug is called a whitehead. If the comedo projects above the pore, it incorporates pigmented skin cells and develops a dark color; it is consequently called a blackhead. Sometimes a follicle becomes so engorged with a plug that it breaks open under the surface of the skin, allowing bacteria to spread and cause an infection called a pimple. Since teen boys produce more androgen than girls do, they tend to have more acne.

Sweat glands in both girls and boys become more active during puberty. Hormones stimulate the production of new chemicals in the body's sweat. Some of these chemicals are pheromones, compounds that are similar in structure to hormones. Pheromones are vitally important to many species of animals because they act as chemical signals to members of the opposite sex. In humans, the roles of pheromones are not completely understood, although research indicates that pheromones released by one person

Height and weight increase dramatically during puberty. The growth spurt begins earlier in girls than boys.

Acne is caused by fluctuations in hormone levels. It appears at puberty and can continue well into adulthood.

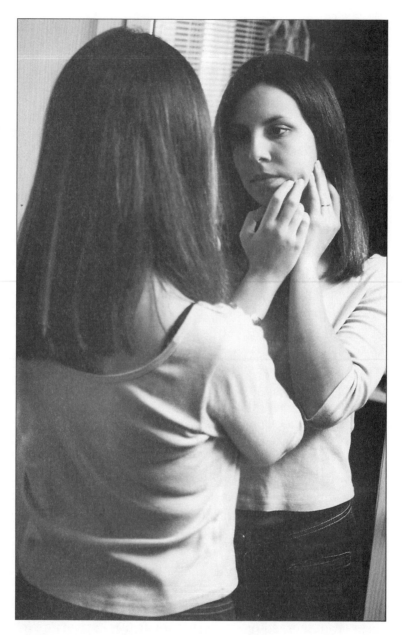

cause changes in the behavior or physical state of another person. One study examined the fact that female college roommates often find themselves menstruating on the same monthly schedule. This research concluded that body odor is the factor that regulated their cycles.

Changes Inside and Out

Just as hormones create alternatives in the way the body looks, they also cause changes inside. The brain, like other organs, must adjust to varying levels of hormones. As a group, young people going through puberty and adolescence are moodier and more emotional than others. Research shows that this volatile behavior is linked to changes in hormone levels. It is not the hormones themselves, but their fluctuations that cause young people to behave inconsistently or inappropriately. By late adolescence, when hormone levels have stabilized, behavior and moods stabilize.

During puberty, many people feel confused by strong emotions that they have not encountered before. For the first time, a young person may experience sexual feelings; these are brought on by changes in levels of sex hormones. Changes in body shape and appearance can cause anxiety. Many of the physical transformations can make young people feel self-conscious about their bodies. And if all parts of the body do not grow and mature on the same schedule, there are likely to be periods of physical awkwardness.

Boys Will Be Boys

Males enter puberty between the ages of ten and fifteen years. One of the first outward changes they undergo is accelerated growth. It is not unusual for a boy to grow as much as four inches in one year. Generally, the hands, feet, and head grow first. The arms and legs, then finally the torso and shoulders eventually catch up.

Like the rest of a boy's body, the larynx and vocal cords grow. As the larynx enlarges, it pushes the Adam's apple forward, making it more prominent in the throat. That is why Adam's apples are more noticeable in adult males than they are in adult females. As this region increases in size, the voice deepens. For a while, the voice may alternate between childhood tones and those of an adult. By late adolescence, it finally stabilizes into its adult tone.

During puberty, the testicles, the organs that make sperm, and the penis, the organ that delivers sperm during sexual intercourse, grow and mature. Inside a boy's body, the internal sexual organs also increase in size. Seminal vesicles, which carry sperm from the testicles to the penis, enlarge. The bulbourethral and Cowper's glands are structures located just below the prostate gland; these three glands play roles in producing seminal fluid.

About a year after penis growth begins, the first night-time ejaculation may occur. Once activated by testosterone, the testes make sperm continuously. A volume of sperm can be stored, but at intervals the stored sperm must be released to make room for new sperm. This can occur automatically as nighttime ejaculation.

Another change is the appearance of hair in new places on the body. Before puberty is over, coarse hair will cover the pubic area, part of the face, and the armpits. Hair growth is stimulated by testosterone. Except for the palms of hands and the soles of the feet, people are covered in hair. Humans have as much hair as apes, but most of it is of the vellus type, which is soft and colorless. At puberty, rising testosterone levels in boys change vellus hair in armpits, around the genitals, and on the face, chest, arms, and legs to a coarser type called terminal hair.

Terminal hair appears in a predictable order. Pubic hair shows up first, followed within a year or two by facial hair. In the beginning, facial hair is only present at the corners of the upper lip. Within months, it can be seen across the lip and then on the upper cheeks. Before the end of puberty, it spreads across the chin and along the lower edges of the face. Underarm hair begins to grow about the same time that facial hair appears. Simultaneously, body hair increases on the legs, arms, and chest.

Some changes occur in the size and shape of the male's breast. During puberty, the area around the nipple, the areola, gets larger, and nipples become more prominent. Some boys develop a slight breast enlargement that includes an increase in fat underneath the nipple. One breast may grow

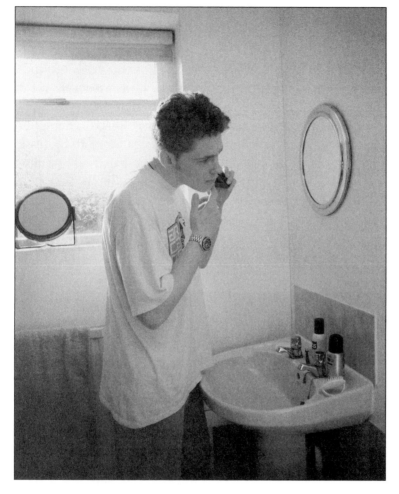

The first sign of facial hair signifies that puberty is almost over.

larger than the other. This condition usually goes away without medical intervention.

What Are Little Girls Made Of?

Girls usually start maturing between eight and thirteen years of age. However, the onset of puberty is affected by nutrition and activity, so girls with low body fat, like athletes, tend to mature later than others. Once the pituitary releases LH and FSH, these two hormones stimulate the ovaries. They, in turn, begin producing another hormone, estrogen. At the same time, the ovaries begin developing mature eggs.

One of the first changes to occur in girls is a period of quick growth, especially in height. Starting at age eight or nine, many girls begin growing and tend to be taller than boys for the next several years. During the years of rapid growth, good nutrition is important. Girls especially need plenty of iron, calcium, and protein in their diets.

The young girl's body also changes shape as it goes through puberty. It becomes curvier because of an increase in the amount of body fat, as well as the pattern of fat distribution. Fat is deposited on the hips and thighs. Some fat is also involved in the development of breasts, which start as "breast buds," small mounds beneath the nipple and areola. As development proceeds, breasts grow rounded and fuller. Initially, one breast may grow faster than the other, but they usually balance out in size before they mature.

Females have as many hair follicles as men, but the small amount of testosterone in their bodies only changes vellus hair in armpits and around genitals to terminal hairs. Pubic hair starts out as a few small strands of terminal hair that slowly increase in number until they form a thick thatch. Pubic and armpit hairs have a course texture, and pubic hair eventually develops curls.

For girls, a milestone in development is the beginning of monthly menstrual cycles. Menarche, the first menstrual period, usually occurs between ages twelve and thirteen, although it is perfectly normal for girls to start as early as nine years of age or as late as sixteen years.

Periods are just a part of the total menstrual cycle. A female is born with thousands of immature eggs in her ovaries. Each month after puberty has begun, some of the eggs in one ovary begin to mature. Eventually, one egg ripens before the others, and it is released from the ovary. This egg travels down an oviduct that connects the ovary to the uterus. The uterus is an organ designed to provide a place for fetal development. If the egg is fertilized by a sperm, it implants in the uterus and grows. In anticipation of receiving a fertilized egg, the uterus develops a thick inner lining of nourishing tissue, plentifully sup-

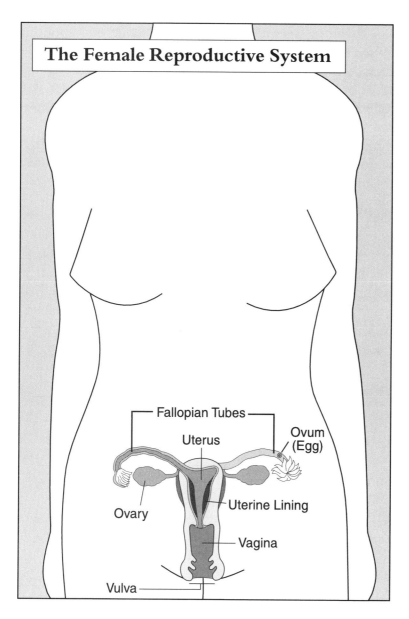

The Female Reproductive System

Fallopian Tubes

Uterus

Ovum (Egg)

Ovary

Uterine Lining

Vagina

Vulva

plied with blood. However, the egg usually is not fertilized. Unfertilized eggs, along with supportive tissue within the uterus, leave the uterus through the vagina. This discharge, called the menstrual flow, lasts from two to seven days. About two weeks later, a new egg is released from an ovary, and the cycle begins again.

The entire menstrual cycle takes about one month. When they begin, periods often occur erratically. However, over time, hormone levels stop fluctuating wildly, and periods appear with more regularity. Generally, menstrual cycles cause little discomfort, although some mild cramping may occur when the uterus expels its inner lining. Between periods, there may be a clear or whitish discharge produced by glands in the vagina that cleanses and moistens this passageway.

Early and Late

Sometimes it is difficult to recognize normal development because puberty appears at different times in different people. However, it is important for physicians and other health care professionals to have some guidelines for defining "normal" so they can have a standard against which to measure any suspected abnormal development. Most practitioners rely on the distribution of pubic hair as a way to determine the stage of puberty. Other traits that can be used are breast size in girls and testicular volume in boys.

Some diseases or conditions can cause atypical puberty, that is, the appearance of secondary sexual characteristics earlier or later than expected. The presence of a growth or tumor on the pituitary, thyroid, or adrenal glands can alter normal sexual development. In girls, the presence of tumors or cysts on the ovaries can affect normal development.

If a young girl develops breasts and pubic hair before age eight, a physician might want to examine her to find out if there is a malfunction in her endocrine system. Only about 30 percent of cases of early puberty in girls reflect a medical disorder. On the other hand, about 50 percent of young boys who experience growth of pubic hair or an increase in testicle size before age nine are suffering from a medical problem.

Disease is also suspected if contrasexual development occurs. If girls show male traits or if boys display feminine features, there may be a problem. Hirsutism, the growth of excessive body hair, may indicate a problem in females of any age, especially young ones.

Ingestion of sex hormones can cause symptoms of early puberty to appear. Hormones in the form of birth control pills can bring about the development of secondary sex characteristics in very young girls. Boys who take androgens, male sex hormones, or anabolic steroids develop too early.

Just as very early puberty may indicate a medical problem, so can delayed puberty. In girls, symptoms of delayed puberty include no pubic hair or development of breast tissue by age fifteen or no menstrual periods for five years after the first appearance of breast tissue. In boys, symptoms are lack of pubic hair and testicular development by age fourteen.

Like early puberty, delayed puberty may have a medical cause, or it may not. The tendency to experience early and late puberty runs in families. If there is no cause, then the condition is labeled "benign," and no treatment is necessary. Eventually, the child falls into normal patterns of development.

One very common cause of delayed puberty is malnutrition. Nutritional deficiencies can be due to a lack of food, a problem for children from families of low socioeconomic class. They can also be due to poor food choices related to eating disorders, use of alcohol or other drugs, or a restrictive weight-loss diet. Not only does poor nutrition delay puberty, but it also has consequences later in life, affecting strength of bones, weight, and final height.

To evaluate either condition, a medical professional may examine blood tests that check levels of hormones, including FSH, LH, estrogen, testosterone, TSH, and thyroxine. If a tumor is suspected, magnetic resonance imaging of the brain and the pituitary can be used to look for it. Normal puberty is a difficult period of change and adjustment, but it can be extremely stressful when development is abnormal. Reassurance from the medical community can often help a young person understand and effectively deal with complications of development.

A Crossroad in Life

The world is brimming with youth who are in the throes of puberty and adolescence. One-sixth of the world's population is made up of young people aged ten to nineteen years. All of these people are experiencing a multitude of physical and mental changes, some of which have a tremendous impact on the health of youth.

Between the ages of eight and fifteen years, a youth leaves childhood and enters puberty, a time of physical maturation. By the end of puberty, the young person will have an adult body that is fully capable of doing its part in the act of reproduction. Puberty and adolescence, a time of mental and social maturation, are the transition periods from childhood to adulthood. During adolescence, young people learn to live and cope with the demands of the world.

Not all teens, of course, survive to adulthood. Thus, examining the way teens die helps explain some of the problems they deal with during life. Accidents cause more deaths in this age group than anything else. The second leading cause of death is homicide, and the third is suicide. Other issues in the lives of youth include alcohol intoxication, substance abuse, depression, sexual experimentation, pregnancy, sexually transmitted diseases, malnutrition, anorexia nervosa, bulimia, and stress. All of these conditions point to attitudes and life-styles that are closely tied to emotions and poor decisions. For young people to find their way to a happy and fulfilling adult life, they need a loving environment in which to mature and lots of adult guidance during the process.

Diseases and Disorders of the Endocrine System

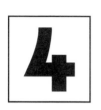

Endocrinology, the study of the endocrine system, is a relatively new field of science. The endocrine system has only been recognized and understood since the early 1900s. However, diseases and disorders that result from an endocrine system gone wrong have been noted for centuries. Ancient paintings and sculptures of the Egyptian ruler Akhenaten portray a man with unusual characteristics. His long slender neck, sharp chin, long arms and fingers, full lips, round hips and thighs, enlarged breasts, and protruding abdomen puzzled historians for centuries. His unusual features were noticed and immortalized by many but understood by none. However, in light of present-day knowledge, his condition is recognizable as an endocrine disorder.

Medical scholars have also identified an array of endocrine ailments alluded to in the Bible. The famous story of the sons of the patriarch Isaac, Esau and his twin brother Jacob, is a classic example. Esau declared that "I am at the point to die" after a day without food. His brother Jacob took advantage of this opportunity to trick the weakened man out of his inheritance; he offered him a bowl of food in exchange for his most precious possession. The two boys were very different. The Bible describes Esau as covered "all over like a hairy garment," whereas Jacob's skin was smooth and hairless. Extreme body hair, associated with faintness due to hunger, is a symptom of an adrenal gland disorder.

Scientists are now able to diagnose and treat endocrine disorders like the one that caused King Akhenaten's unusual shape.

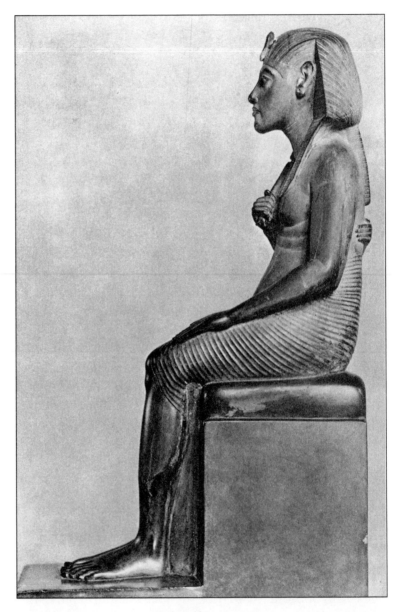

The term "eunuch" appears twenty-six times in the King James version of the New Testament. Eunuchoidism, a condition in which men lack testosterone and therefore do not develop male sexual characteristics, can occur at birth. Testosterone production can be thwarted by dysfunction of the testes or by lack of gonadatrophic hormones, FSH and

LH. More than two thousand years ago, Jesus recognized that some eunuchs "were so born from their mother's womb." It can also be caused by surgical removal of the testicles before puberty.

Modern-day scientists know that when endocrine glands do not function correctly, the concentration of hormones in the blood can become abnormally high or low, resulting in disruption of body functions. Oversecretion of a hormone, or a product of a hormone, is generally described with the prefix *hyper*, as in hyperthyroidism. The prefix that indicates low secretion, or underproduction, is *hypo*, as in hypoglycemia. All of the endocrine glands are subject to disease or injury that can result in hypo- or hypersecretion. Problems associated with the pituitary gland are the most common type.

Glandular Growth Disorders

The pituitary gland has several vital functions. In the anterior lobe, it manufactures hormones that switch on other endocrine glands, as well as growth hormone and prolactin. The posterior lobe stores antidiuretic hormone and oxytocin. Several complications result from over- or undersecretion of any of these hormones. Two of the most noticeable endocrine disorders result from hyperpituitarism, or the secretion of too much growth hormone. Normally, growth hormone is produced abundantly until adulthood. At that time, the pituitary slows its production of the hormone, and growth slows or stops. The kind of damage done by an overactive pituitary depends on the time in life when the gland begins to malfunction.

During childhood and puberty, bones in the legs and arms grow, eventually reaching their full adult size between the ages of eighteen and twenty-one. If the pituitary gland releases too much growth hormone during this growing phase, bones continue to grow longer than they should. As a result, some individuals grow as tall as nine feet, a condition known as gigantism. People who suffer from this disorder usually experience other health problems, such as diabetes and incomplete sexual development. Although most reach full mental development, a few suffer mental retardation. Gigantism is most often caused by a tumor on the pituitary. The presence of a growth on the pituitary gland puts pressure on neighboring brain tissues, such as the optic nerve, causing visual problems and headaches. In some cases, the tumor destroys the entire pituitary gland. Without the hormones produced by this master gland, death is inevitable.

When a person reaches adulthood, normal production of growth hormone slows, and long bones stop growing. However, if the pituitary begins producing high levels of growth hormone during adulthood, it causes bones to enlarge and deform in a condition called acromegaly. The onset of this disorder is subtle, and it is often not diagnosed until middle age. Bones of the hands, feet, and face are especially affected. Excess growth hormone also stimulates enlargement and swelling of soft tissues. Skin over the entire body, especially the face, takes on a very coarse appearance because oil and sweat glands enlarge, often producing offensive body odor. The nose and lips enlarge and the jaw assumes a sharp, protruding shape. Joint pain often accompanies changes in bone structure, and after many years it can develop into crippling arthritis. Many acromegalics have curved spines that force them to walk in a bent position. Headaches and impaired vision are other symptoms commonly found in this disorder. The hearts of people afflicted with acromegaly may enlarge and lose their ability to function properly, ultimately causing heart failure. Overproduction of growth hormone is usually due to a benign, or noncancerous, tumor of the pituitary gland. Like any tumor on the gland, it compresses nearby tissues in the brain. Treatment usually requires removal of the tumor through surgery or with radiation therapy.

Hypopituitarism, or undersecretion of hormones by the pituitary gland, can result in small size or dwarfism in extreme cases. A child who lacks sufficient quantities of

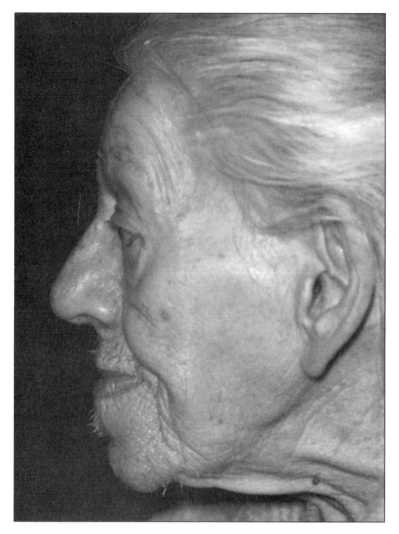

The jutting jaw and long face are signs of acromegaly, a condition that results from too much growth hormone during adulthood.

growth hormone is often smaller than other children the same age and shows much slower rates of growth. Typically, these small children have a chubby body build and a round face. Since growth of all body parts is slow, the limbs are proportionate to the head and torso, unlike in some other forms of dwarfism in which the arms and legs are disproportionately short. At the age of ten years, a child suffering from lack of growth hormone has the body size of an average five year old. At twenty years, the body size is about the same as that of a seven year old.

Lack of growth hormone may be due to an injury to the pituitary gland; it is more likely, however, that a tumor on the pituitary is the cause. If a tumor presses on other areas of the brain as well, surgical removal is necessary. Injections of supplemental growth hormone, varying from one a week to three or four each week, for several years, are then required. Such treatment usually results in a quick increase in the growth rate. Conditions that cause a lack of growth hormone often cause a lack of other pituitary hormones, so supplements of thyroid hormone, cortisol, and sex hormones may also be needed.

Other Pituitary Problems

Another, and more common, type of tumor found on the pituitary is a prolactinoma. This benign growth causes the production of too much prolactin. Like other benign growths, the tumor may exert pressure on surrounding brain tissue, creating headaches and visual problems. In women, a prolactinoma can cause changes in the normal menstrual cycle. Non-nursing women may develop milk in their breasts. Loss of libido, or interest in sex, is also commonly reported by women. Men often suffer from impotence. In both sexes, treatment generally includes removal of the tumor.

A relatively rare disease named diabetes insipidus, to distinguish it from the better known condition diabetes mellitus, can result if the pituitary does not produce adequate amounts of antidiuretic hormone. The name for this condition is appropriate because, in Latin, diabetes means "increased urine output." Symptoms of diabetes insipidus include a thirst so enormous that people drink large volumes of water, some up to forty quarts each day. Excessive water intake increases the volume of urine. As a result, most of the water taken into the body is lost, so a person with diabetes insipidus is chronically dehydrated, no matter how much water he or she drinks. This condition can result if the hypothalamus produces too little or if the pituitary does not release enough antidiuretic hormone. Treatment includes supplements of the hormone.

Trouble with the Thyroid and Parathyroid Glands

A goiter is a swelling on the neck that results from an abnormal enlargement of the thyroid gland. At one time, so many people in the Midwest had goiter that the area became known as the "goiter belt." Research eventually showed that the soil in the Midwest is low in iodine, an element that the thyroid needs to make hormones. Iodine is usually supplied in the diet, so people living on iodine-poor soil are missing an essential nutrient. When the body sends a signal to the thyroid gland for thyroid

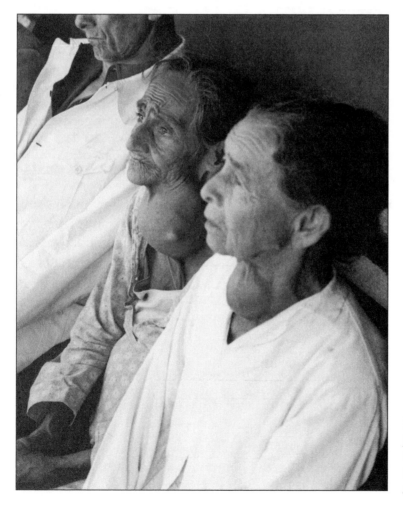

These women suffer from goiters, an abnormal enlargement of the thyroid gland.

hormones, the gland tries to manufacture them. Even though the requested hormones cannot be made without iodine, the gland keeps trying to fill the orders. As a result, the thyroid gland swells and produces a goiter in the neck.

The thyroid cannot function unless it is activated by thyroid-stimulating hormone (TSH). Any health problem that reduces the normal output of TSH also reduces the production of thyroid hormones. Thyroid hormones are essential to normal physical and mental development. Cretinism is a condition that develops if undersecretion occurs during fetal development, infancy, or childhood. Immediately after birth, a child born with no thyroid function appears to be normal because the fetus received thyroid hormones from its mother. However, within a few weeks, physical and mental growth slows. The face of a child afflicted with cretinism becomes misshapen and is characterized by a broad nose, small eyes, puffy eyelids, and a tongue that protrudes from the mouth. Without treatment, this condition results in mental retardation and dwarfism. If the problem is diagnosed very early, thyroxine can be given in therapeutic doses, avoiding the onset of symptoms.

If hypothyroidism occurs in adulthood, symptoms are different. Lack of thyroid hormones in adults results in myxedema, a condition that causes mental and physical sluggishness. Symptoms include fatigue, muscle weakness, slow heart rate, low body temperature, and weight gain. A person suffering from myxedema may sleep fourteen to sixteen hours a day. Thyroxine supplements can compensate for the lack of these hormones in the body and alleviate many of the symptoms.

Overproduction of thyroid hormones, hyperthyroidism, usually results from a tumor on the thyroid gland. Symptoms are just the opposite of those of hypothyroidism; they include rapid heart rate, agitated or hyperactive behavior, and weight loss. Graves' disease is one form of hyperthyroidism. A person with Graves' disease has a very characteristic appearance: the facial expression is tense, and the eyes

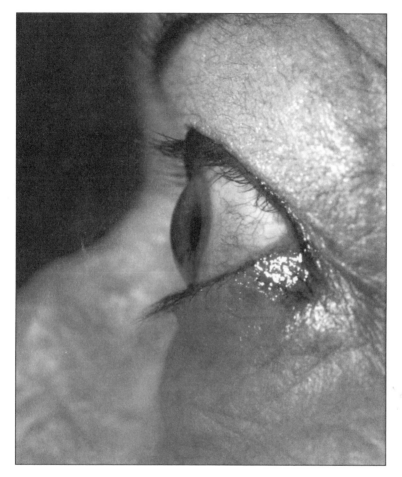

The bulging eyes of Graves' disease can lead to double vision and difficulty moving and closing the eyes.

bulge because of swelling of tissue in the eye sockets. In cases of severe bulging, the eyelids cannot close, and the optic nerve is damaged by pressure from the tumor. Always hungry, a person with Graves' disease eats excessively but still loses weight because the food's energy is burned up abnormally fast. Usually, Graves' disease is caused by an autoimmune disorder in which the body attacks its own thyroid gland, stimulating it to overactivity. Removal of some of the gland is a common treatment.

The parathyroid glands, tiny structures located on the thyroid, are also subject to malfunction. In hyperparathyroidism, one or more overactive parathyroid glands secrete too much parathyroid hormone, causing blood calcium levels to rise. In mild cases, the symptoms are often slight and not very specific: weakness, fatigue, depression, and aches. However, excessive calcium in the blood signals to a doctor that something may be wrong. In severe cases, symptoms are more obvious and include nausea, vomiting, constipation, confusion, and increased thirst and urination. The condition can also cause kidney stones, thinning of bones, high blood pressure, and stomach ulcers. Hyperparathyroidism is usually caused by a benign tumor of the gland. Ninety-five percent of the time, surgical removal of the gland solves the problem.

Adrenal Ailments

Like other endocrine glands, the adrenals are subject to malfunction. Addison's disease develops when the adrenal cortexes do not produce enough cortisol and aldosterone. The cause of Addison's is usually unknown, although a small number of cases result from cancer or an infection with tuberculosis. Symptoms of Addison's disease include weakness, fatigue, dizziness, and an inability to tolerate cold temperatures. The skin often takes on a bronze color, and purple or black discoloration may occur around the lips and in areas where skin bends or folds, such as the inside of the elbows. Symptoms develop slowly, so they may not be noticed immediately. However, a stressful situation, like an illness or accident, can make symptoms worse. During an addisonian crisis, one can experience severe problems such as penetrating low back pain, vomiting, diarrhea, low blood pressure, and loss of consciousness. The most common cause of Addison's disease is destruction of the adrenals by the body's own immune system. Treatment includes supplements of corticosteroids and aldosterone.

Just as hyposecretion causes Addison's disease, hypersecretion of the adrenal can also cause problems. Overproduction of adrenal hormones is most often caused by tumors. A tumor in the adrenal medulla brings about the production of too much aldosterone. Consequently, the body retains water and sodium, causing tissues to swell and blood pressure to rise. High levels of aldosterone also set in motion excessive loss of potassium, damaging the activity of the heart and the nervous system.

A tumor in the adrenal cortex can lead to Cushing's syndrome. In Cushing's syndrome the body makes too much cortisol. Elevated levels of this hormone cause high blood pressure, bone damage, depression of the immune system, and diabetes. Other consequences of Cushing's syndrome include a rounding of the face and the appearance of a "buffalo hump" of fat on the upper back. Skin becomes thin and bruises easily, and fat accumulates on the abdomen, buttocks, and breasts. Muscles lose their strength and no longer maintain muscle tone. Treatment is generally surgical removal of the gland, followed by administration of replacement hormones.

Adrenogenital syndrome, like Cushing's syndrome, is caused by oversecretion by an endocrine gland. In this case, the adrenal produces too much androgen, the male hormone. Higher than normal levels of androgen in either females or young males can cause masculinization, or the appearance of male traits. In females and boys, high levels of androgens cause excessive body or facial hair, balding on the top of the head, deepening of the voice, thickening of the skin, and an increase in muscle size. Young males rapidly develop secondary sex characteristics, including growth of sexual organs and feelings of sexual desire. In adult males, the symptoms may be obscured by the normal male traits, making diagnosis difficult. The cause of adrenal oversecretion is usually a tumor, and treatment may require removal of the gland.

Pancreas on Strike

One of the most common endocrine diseases is diabetes mellitus, a condition in which blood levels of glucose are abnormally high. Some symptoms of diabetes are frequent urination, abnormal thirst, hunger, drowsiness, nausea, decreased endurance, and susceptibility to infections. The term *mellitus*, which means "honey" in Latin, aptly describes the sweetness of a diabetic's urine, the result of too much blood sugar in the body. Glucose builds up in the blood if the islets of Langerhans in the pancreas do not make sufficient insulin or if body cells cannot use insulin to take in glucose. In either case, as the kidneys filter blood, they cannot reabsorb all of the sugar, and some of it becomes part of the urine. Moreover, because

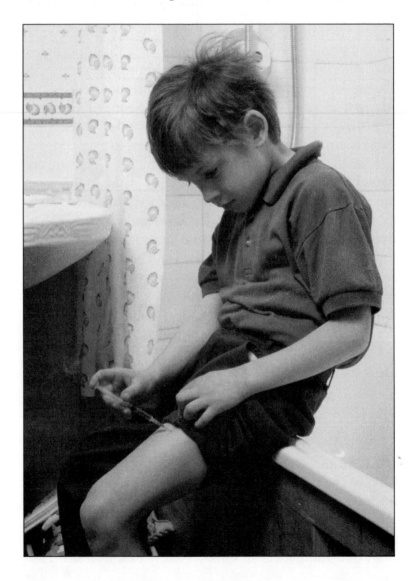

A young boy with Type I diabetes injects insulin.

glucose acts as a diuretic, as it is lost from the body, water follows, hence the frequent urination that is typical of this disease.

A severe form of the disease, called Type I or insulin-dependent diabetes, occurs before age twenty. It is caused by the body's attack on its own insulin-secreting cells; eventually the pancreatic cells are destroyed. Type I, which accounts for about 15 percent of all cases of diabetes, requires injections or infusions of insulin throughout the day to regulate glucose levels, as well as a food and exercise plan. The kind of diabetes that begins in adulthood is called Type II or non-insulin-dependent diabetes. It is caused by the loss of insulin receptors on cells, preventing insulin from transporting glucose into cells. Treatment includes a careful diet that avoids the types of foods that produce a lot of insulin. Exercise and weight control are also important in the management of Type II diabetes.

Whereas levels of blood sugar are higher than normal in diabetes, they are too low in another condition, hypoglycemia. When blood sugar levels begin to fall, the body naturally responds by releasing adrenaline. This hormone stimulates the release of sugar from body stores. It also causes feelings related to stress, such as faintness, sweating, nervousness, and mental confusion. Symptoms of hypoglycemia usually begin gradually, but they can suddenly progress from mild discomfort to total confusion within a few minutes. Without treatment, severe cases can result in coma, convulsions, and death. If a hypoglycemic person is conscious, he or she is encouraged to eat. However, if the person is unconscious, injections of glucose may be needed. Severe hypoglycemia can be due to a tumor in the pancreas.

Pineal Gland Puzzlers

Like the seasons, tides, and many other systems in nature, the body operates in regular cycles. Many body functions, such as sleep and wakefulness, body temperature, and the pulse, follow the same rhythm. Light is one of the factors that helps these rhythms beat together.

Light reaches the brain through the eye. After striking the retina, light travels along nerves in the eye to an area of the hypothalamus that controls the pineal gland. The pineal gland secretes the hormone melatonin, which helps regulate normal rhythms of sleep and wakefulness. Melatonin production is slowed by light.

Mood is also affected by light and production of melatonin. Moods seem to have seasonal rhythms. Many people feel better in the summer and more anxious or depressed in the winter. The moods of people who suffer from seasonal affective disorder (SAD) are greatly exaggerated. In the fall, as days grow shorter, people with SAD have trouble sleeping and they feel very anxious. Treatment with bright light for two hours a day can help to minimize these symptoms.

Disorders of the Sex Organs

The sex organs can suffer from disorders that affect their normal production of male and female hormones. An abnormal increase in the function of gonads causes hypergonadism. In males, this condition is usually the result of a tumor of the testes. The resulting overproduction of testosterone causes the growing ends of bones to fuse too early in life, so true adult height is not reached. Hypergonadism is rare in females.

Hypogonadism, or undersecretion by the gonads, afflicts the sexes with equal frequency. There are several scenarios that can lead to hypogonadism in males. If the testes do not descend in childhood, they shrink and fail to produce the male hormone, testosterone. Testes may fail to develop because they are not properly stimulated by gonadotropic hormones from the pituitary. In either case, secondary male characteristics are lacking. Surgical removal of male gonads before puberty causes the same symptoms. However, if the testes are removed after puberty, not all secondary male sexual characteristics are lost. In these cases, supplements of testosterone help maintain them.

In females, hypogonadism may be due to a lack of ovaries or poorly formed ovaries. When ovaries are not present, or if they are lost before puberty, female eunuchism results. Such females have no secondary sexual characteristics, and their sexual organs do not mature. Lack of female hormones causes excessive growth of long bones, so women suffering from this condition are extremely tall. If the ovaries are lost to disease or surgically removed after sexual maturity is reached, the uterus shrinks, the vagina becomes smaller, the breasts lose some of their supporting fat, and the pubic hair thins. These are the same characteristics that appear after menopause, the point at which the ovaries normally stop functioning.

Ailments and Afflictions

The endocrine system affects every cell in the body. Secretions of endocrine glands help determine mental abilities, as well as physical characteristics such as height, agility, and appearance. Many aspects of behavior, especially those related to sexual urges, are ruled by endocrine glands. Therefore, it makes sense that imbalances within the endocrine system cause a wide variety of problems.

Endocrine disorders have been with man since the beginning of time. Captured in art, literature, history, and sociology, the symptoms of many disorders are obvious. The biblical warrior Goliath may have been a textbook case of gigantism. Because of his disorder, he most likely suffered from complications such as diabetes and poor vision. It could have been his lack of keen vision that made it difficult for him to see the small flying missile that was his demise. On the other extreme, court jesters, dwarfs who kept company with the leaders of the world, are well known in history. Another group of very short people are the pygmies of Africa, who share a genetic condition that interferes with growth hormone's ability to lengthen bones.

Less than one hundred years ago, physicians did not understand the nature of endocrine glands and therefore could not determine the causes of endocrine disorders. Consequently, conditions such as diabetes insipidus, diabetes mellitus, and cretinism resulted in death. Today, most disorders of the endocrine system can be medically managed. Some, such as stunted growth due to lack of growth hormone, can even be prevented.

High-Tech Help for Endocrine Ailments

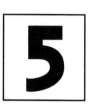

The endocrine glands produce, or play a role in producing, hormones, chemicals that regulate body functions. For this reason the diagnosis and treatment of disorders of the endocrine glands are very important to a person's quality and quantity of life. Because of ongoing research, today many endocrine disorders can be successfully diagnosed.

When John F. Kennedy ran for office in 1960, he knew he had Addison's disease. His adrenal glands no longer functioned, and his health depended entirely on hormone replacement therapy, which did not exist until the early 1900s. Had Kennedy been born sixty years earlier, he would not have been able to live as actively as he did in the fifth decade of his life. Advancements made in recent years improve the lives of endocrine-challenged people. Diagnosis and treatment of all endocrine disorders begin with a thorough examination. One of the most common glands to present problems is the thyroid.

Diagnosing Thyroid Disorders

When doctors detect unusual lumps or growths in a patient's neck near the thyroid gland, they generally order a series of tests to evaluate the abnormality. A thyroid scan and a radioactive iodine uptake (RAIU) test are usually performed. These two procedures, which were among the first nuclear scans introduced into medicine, are

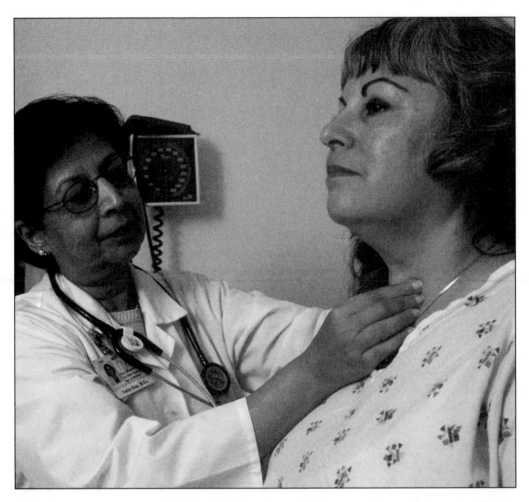

A doctor performs a common test for thyroid disorders. She feels a patient's neck for lumps or other abnormalities.

sometimes performed at the same time so that physicians can evaluate both the structure and the function of the thyroid.

Before either test, the patient is given a radioactive substance called a tracer. The radioactive isotope can be administered orally by drink or pill, or it can be injected into the bloodstream. Once the tracer is in the body, the thyroid gland begins absorbing it from the bloodstream. As radioactive tracer collects in the thyroid gland, a series of pictures is made.

The pictures result from one of two techniques: a camera scan or a computerized rectilinear thyroid (CRT) scan. The camera scan is most commonly employed. It utilizes a special camera that can show views of the entire thyroid gland. The CRT, on the other hand, employs a computer to improve the clarity of camera scan pictures and to measure thyroid size. The ability of the CRT to provide accurate sizing of the thyroid helps the physician determine if the gland is growing or decreasing in size when follow-up scans are made.

After the isotope has been given time to accumulate in the thyroid gland, the patient is asked to recline on a movable table. The patient's neck and chest are carefully positioned under the scanner camera. As the patient lies still, the scanner detects the location and intensity of the radioactive rays being emitted by the isotope.

Information produced about the shape, size, and location of the thyroid gland during the scan gives the physician many clues about the health of the gland. If the thyroid is enlarged or pushed to one side, a tumor may be present. Regions of the thyroid that are not functioning normally cannot take up the isotope and will appear as "cold" spots on the scan. Healthy thyroid tissue has a uniform gray color. Nodules appear either lighter or darker than the thyroid, depending on the amount of iodine they absorbed. Tumors and other areas of dysfunction are usually lighter in color.

The radioactive iodine uptake test evaluates thyroid function by measuring the percentage of radioactive iodine that has been taken up by the gland. After the patient is given a dose of radioactive iodine, usually in pill form, there is a twenty-four-hour wait to allow some of the iodine to be concentrated in the thyroid gland; the remainder will be eliminated from the body through urination. The amount of iodine concentrated in the thyroid gland is measured by a special probe to see if the quantity absorbed from the bloodstream for the manufacture of thyroid hormone is within normal levels. Overactive glands generally have a higher rate of uptake than underactive glands. The information obtained from the RAIU helps physicians calculate the amount and type of medication needed to treat an overactive gland.

Other tests that may be used along with the thyroid scan include blood work and such imaging techniques as ultrasound and CT scans. Blood work reveals chemical imbalances within the body, such as elevated or lowered levels of hormones. Ultrasound and CT images help to visualize any unusual growth. If an abnormal growth is located, a small section of it may be surgically removed for microscopic evaluation to determine whether or not cancer is involved.

Checking Out the Parathyroid Glands

The parathryroid glands, small nodules on the thyroid, can be sites of tumors that cause devastating health challenges. When these tiny glands malfunction, they may need to be surgically removed. Usually only one of the four parathyroid glands goes wrong, and it is critical that doctors remove the defective gland instead of a healthy one. This is a challenging task because a parathyroid is about the size of a grain of rice.

In the past, ultrasound and CT were the only techniques available for locating these glands. Even with these imagers, the extremely small parathyroids were hard to locate. Help arrived in the early 1990s in the form of the Sestamibi scan. This technology quickly became the preferred method of evaluating parathyroid health.

Sestamibi is the name of a protein that can be labeled with a radioactive tracer, technetium 99. Sestamibi and its attached technetium 99, a safe, low-dose radioactive substance, can be injected into a patient's vein. Normally, parathyroid glands are inactive; they do not have anything to do when calcium levels in the blood are appropriate. Consequently, normal parathyroids do not absorb and retain the technetium. However, an abnormal parathyroid gland functions at inappropriate times and will absorb the radioactive element. A scanning camera, which operates very much like a Geiger counter, is placed over the patient's neck to pick up radiation emitted by the malfunctioning gland. The camera's electronic processors interpret the data and display the information as an image on a monitor. Normal parathyroid glands are not seen on the image since they do not pick up the radioactive material.

After the diseased parathyroid is pinpointed, patients requiring surgery are often sent to a same-day surgery center for removal of the gland. The procedure takes no more than thirty minutes. If surgery is done on the same day the radioisotope is given to the patient, the surgeon can use the radiation to determine where to make an incision in the neck. A pencil-like gamma ray detector probe held over the neck will home in on the location of the parathyroid. This helps surgeons make their incisions without guesswork.

Keeping Diabetes in Check

Scientists know that keeping the blood glucose level under control is essential to lowering the risks associated with diabetes, which include vascular disease such as damage to blood vessels and loss of circulation, nerve damage, loss of vision, and kidney failure. Therefore, many people who suffer from diabetes monitor their blood glucose levels every day. At-home monitoring kits help diabetics determine whether or not they are taking their medication at the most appropriate dosage.

Glucose monitors have improved since they were first introduced to the market. Early versions required users to prick their fingers to produce a small drop of blood. The drop was applied to the test strip; then after one minute the user wiped away excess blood with a cotton ball. Within thirty seconds or so the strip with the dried blood had to be inserted into the monitor, which digitally displayed the glucose levels. The newer at-home glucose monitors do not require strict timing and usually have other simplifying features.

Most at-home glucose monitors weigh only a few ounces and are about the size of a calculator. The kits are made up of a battery-operated monitor and test strips. A drop of

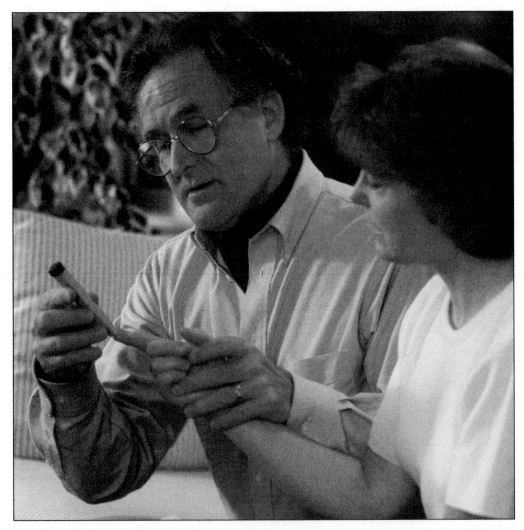

A diabetic has her glucose level checked. Diabetics must monitor their glucose levels to determine the most appropriate time and dosage for their medication.

blood is placed on a test strip, which is then inserted into the monitor. The newest models rely on electrical current to measure the blood glucose level on the test strips. Recently, diabetics have been offered a noninvasive way to keep a constant check on their glucose levels. A new device, the GlucoWatch Biographer, made by Cygnus, Inc., of Redwood, California, received approval from the Food and Drug Administration (FDA) on March 22, 2001, for public use in America. The GlucoWatch Biographer, worn like a wristwatch, consists of a monitor (the

Biographer) that contains a small disposable pad (an Auto Sensor) beneath it to absorb fluid from the diabetic's skin.

The GlucoWatch Biographer is currently being used along with the traditional finger prick tests to serve as a supplemental way for diabetics to check glucose levels. The watch functions by emitting a low electrical current that pulls glucose through the skin into the disposable pad on the underside of the watch. As the glucose is collected on the pad, the autosensor converts it into an electrical signal that is displayed on the monitor as a glucose reading. The GlucoWatch also creates an electronic diary of past readings so the user can review recent trends in glucose readings. In the future, such a monitor may prove to be reliable enough to eliminate finger prick tests.

No More Shots

By monitoring their blood glucose levels, diabetics can determine whether or not they need supplements of insulin. Armed with this lifesaving information, many people give themselves one or more injections each day. Unfortunately for some, insulin injections do not solve all of their problems. People who suffer extreme fluctuations in sugar, especially at night or after strenuous exercise when sugar levels plummet, need a more constant supply of the hormone. In the last decade, the insulin pump has been developed to offer an alternative to daily or more frequent shots.

The insulin pump consists of a pump unit and a part called an infusion set. The pump unit is encased in a plastic container about the size of a deck of cards. Inside the pump unit is a cartridge containing several days' worth of insulin, a small battery-operated pump, and a computer chip to regulate the amount of insulin administered. The infusion set, simply a thin plastic tube with a fine needle at one end, carries insulin from the pump to the diabetic.

To use the insulin pump, the diabetic inserts the needle of the infusion set under the skin of the abdomen, thigh, or buttocks. Every two or three days, the infusion set must be removed and a new one inserted. This can be done manually or with an automatic insertion device. The small pump unit is carried with a clip on the user's waistband, much like a pager.

To keep blood glucose levels within the desired range between meals and overnight, the pump delivers small amounts of insulin twenty-four hours a day according to a programmed plan that the user enters into the pump. When the diabetic eats, a larger dose can be sent to the bloodstream to match the amount of food consumed. The pump does not automatically check blood glucose, so the user still monitors his or her level. However, instead of taking an insulin shot if one is needed, the user simply presses a button to specify the insulin amount, and the pump administers that volume of insulin into the bloodstream.

The type of insulin used in the pump is different from that used in injections. The pumps use a fast-acting form that takes effect in the body within a matter of only ten to twenty minutes. This allows diabetics to quickly learn if the values they programmed into the pump unit are right for them.

A New Supply of Islet Cells

In the United States alone there are over one million people with juvenile diabetes, a disease that results when the body lacks the insulin-producing islet cells of the pancreas. Some of these Type I diabetics can effectively control their disease with supplements of insulin, but others are not so lucky. In some diabetics, blood glucose levels are extremely hard to control, causing repeated episodes of very high or very low blood sugar. On the other hand, some diabetics are able to keep their blood levels in normal ranges but still suffer the vascular and nerve complications that go with the disease. For these two groups, pancreatic islet cell transplants may provide a solution.

This new procedure, still in the experimental stages, transplants islet cells from a donor pancreas into the body of a diabetic. Once implanted, the pancreatic islet cells begin to make and release insulin. Although scientists have been studying this process for the last twenty-five years, it was Dr. James Shapiro at the University of Alberta in Edmonton, Canada, who successfully freed eight diabetics from insulin injections in 1999. Dr. Shapiro's technique, called the Edmonton Protocol, transplants islet cells into the large vein of the liver. Shapiro's researchers remove the islet cells from the pancreas of a deceased donor.

The transplant, which requires only local anesthesia, is not a major surgical procedure and takes less than an hour

Scientists display human islet cells on a monitor. Islet cell transplant is an experimental procedure that might help diabetics.

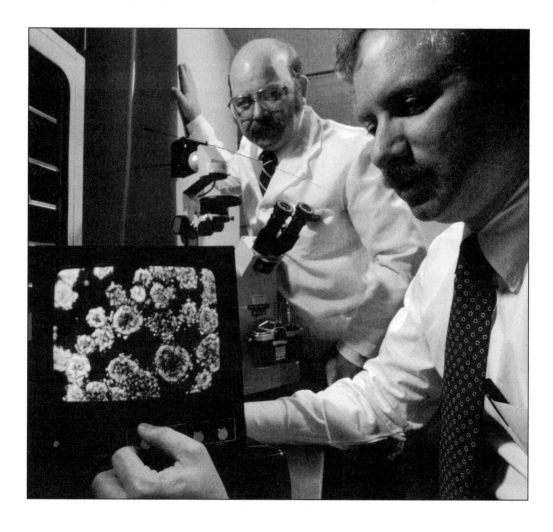

to complete. The surgeon makes a small incision in the upper abdomen of the patient and then uses ultrasound imaging to guide a plastic catheter through the incision and into the liver. Once the catheter is in place, the islet cells are delivered to the liver via the catheter.

After surgery, the patient needs medications to prevent islet cell rejection by the immune system. Since rejection is a huge problem in all types of transplants, immunosuppressant drugs are very important. However, these medications depress the entire immune system, putting the patient more at risk for infectious diseases than the general population.

Since this procedure is still in its experimental stages, scientists do not know the long-term effects of islet cell transplants. It will take another twenty or thirty years to determine whether the transplanted cells will lose their effectiveness over time and whether the transplants have been more than temporarily successful.

The Pituitary Prognosis

The pituitary gland, about the size of a pea, is nestled beneath the brain. This very important gland both produces and controls a variety of hormones. When abnormal growths occur on the small gland, they often have to be surgically removed. Any disorder in or near the brain can be difficult to treat. Surgical removal of growths within the brain requires much expertise to avoid damaging the surrounding tissues.

Traditionally, surgeons have operated on the pituitary gland by making an incision under the upper lip or nostril. After the first incision, surgeons dissected the tissue in the middle nose to clear a path through the sphenoid bone and up to the base of the skull. After reaching the pituitary, surgeons used a microscope-tipped instrument to look through the newly created corridor. This setup allowed them to locate and then carefully remove the tumor from the pituitary gland. During this tedious operation, surgeons had to be careful to avoid injuring the carotid artery and optic nerve. Even so, the procedure sometimes left patients with both cosmetic defects and functional disabilities.

A new technique of removing some pituitary tumors involves the use of a tiny endoscope. This viewing device, contained in a tube about twenty centimeters long, is introduced into the nostril of the patient, eliminating the need to cut through the lip, nose, and brain tissue. Once inside the nostril, the endoscope allows the surgeon to view the gland and area surrounding it. With the gland in sight, the surgeon can deal with the pituitary tumor without disturbing the brain itself. Once the endoscope is positioned to give the best view of the pituitary gland, surgeons pass dissection instruments through the endoscope to remove the tumor.

The pituitary gland itself, along with the human growth hormone (HGH) it produces, has been on the technological newsfront since the 1970s. Children whose bodies do not secrete enough HGH experience stunted growth. After adolescence the human body produces less HGH. As people age, the amount of HGH continues to decline, accounting for the increase in fat and the reduction in lean body mass in older adults.

The first treatment designed for children suffering from HGH deficiency consisted of a series of injections of the growth hormone that had been taken from the brains of cadavers. The injections usually helped children with stunted growth to mature at a normal rate. However, between 1958 and 1980, some of the children in treatment died of a neurological disorder called Creutzfeldt-Jakob disease (CJD). The virus causing CJD, which has many of the same symptoms as "mad cow disease," was being transmitted through the growth hormone injections made from the cadavers. Since growth hormone loses its effectiveness if heated, there was no way to kill the virus. The Food and Drug Administration intervened and put an immediate end to these growth hormone injections.

Early work with cadaver HGH made it clear that children with HGH deficiencies could benefit from a safe, artificial form of the hormone, if one could be created. To this end, scientists had to isolate HGH and then study the genetic make-up of the protein. In 1979, scientists used recombinant DNA technology to create a form of growth hormone in the laboratory, and by 1985 the genetically engineered growth hormone was placed on the American market.

To genetically engineer HGH, the gene that produces HGH was isolated from cells and then added to the genes of specially selected strains of bacteria. Once a gene is incorporated into the genetic material of bacteria, the bacterial cells activate that gene. As a result, the bacteria manufacture that gene's products, just as they make products from their own genes. In the case of the HGH gene, the product is HGH. In a laboratory, large quantities of the modified bacteria are grown in a specialized medium. They are then killed and opened so the growth hormone can be extracted and purified.

Advances in Adrenal Treatments

The adrenal glands can be the sites of tumors and diseases. Some tumors that grow on the adrenal glands can cause excess hormone to be secreted. Even noncancerous tumors of the adrenal gland can result in the secretion of large quantities of aldosterone. When this occurs, the salt balance of the blood is disrupted, causing symptoms such as high blood pressure, high levels of sodium in the serum, and low levels of potassium. In these cases, the adrenal gland itself must be removed.

Like other surgeries of the endocrine gland, adrenal gland surgery was once a major operation that required long incisions and lengthy recovery times. Today, removal of the adrenal gland, a procedure called an adrenalectomy, can be performed by laparoscopic surgery if the tumor is small or known to be benign. Laparoscopic surgery for adrenal gland removal was developed in the middle 1990s and has become the operation of choice whenever possible for an adrenalectomy.

In the laparoscopic procedure, the patient is anesthetized, and the surgeon makes a series of small incisions in the abdomen for the insertion of specialized instruments needed to perform the operation. One of the instruments pumps air into the abdominal cavity to separate the intestines and other organs from the tissues being examined. After the abdomen is inflated, the laparoscopic camera is placed inside one of the incisions to give the surgeon a view of the surgical site to monitor his progress. The remaining incisions provide entrance ways for other instruments such as scissors and forceps.

Once the camera has been put in place, the surgeon begins to remove the malfunctioning gland, which must be carefully separated from the kidney on which it rests. It also must be teased away from connections to the spleen and pancreas. Like a submarine captain navigating with the aid of a periscope, the surgeon views the site through a laparoscopic camera. With narrow instruments inserted through tiny surgical slits, the surgeon lifts the pancreas and spleen away from the adrenal gland. Before the severed, tumor-bearing gland is taken from the body, it is placed in a small cloth bag inserted through one of the incision sites.

The Endocrine Control System

A body cannot function without its endocrine system, the communication center that broadcasts chemical messages needed to sustain life in the body. Through complex signals, endocrine glands control reproduction, growth, and development. They determine whether a person is short or tall, strong or weak. Endocrine glands decide whether one copes well with stress or rages and lashes out when faced with dangers, fears, and anxiety.

As the power behind development, the endocrine system regulates levels of hormones coursing through the body. Through signals from the brain and feedback from the body, it precisely orchestrates the flood of chemical changes that tell a young body to grow, change, and mature. It provides males with the characteristics of sexually reproductive men, as well as those that make boys look like men. Likewise, endocrine secretions are in charge of the metamorphosis that converts little girls into women capable of carrying and nourishing new life.

When the endocrine system malfunctions, its effects are often obvious and detrimental. Historical literature has preserved information about the lives of thousands of individuals whose endocrine systems did not work to perfection: eunuchs, dwarfs, giants, acromegalics, diabetics, and hypoglycemics. Those whose endocrine systems failed them entirely were not recorded in historical records because their lives were fleeting and death came quickly.

Since the early 1900s, scientists have sought to understand the endocrine system and all of the ramifications of its

Miniature instruments are inserted through a laparoscopic tube and operated outside the body. Laparoscopic surgery results in faster recovery and fewer complications.

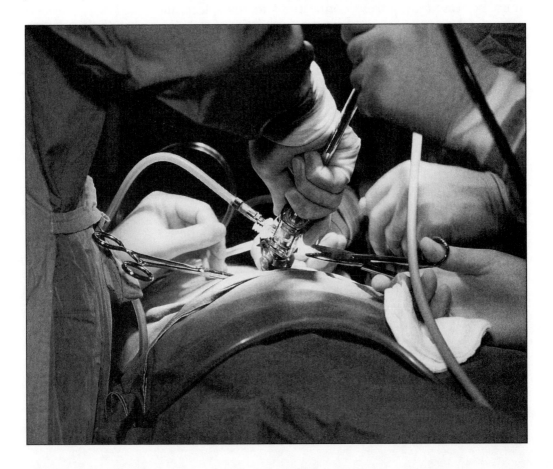

influence. Because of the successes of medical research, doctors are now able to treat many of the conditions that were once debilitating or fatal.

The advances of medicine have enabled doctors to improve the quality of life for millions of individuals, especially those with diabetes. The future looks bright for many afflicted with endocrine challenges, and there is good news emerging every day from laboratories involved in the continuing research.

GLOSSARY

adrenaline: Epinephrine; primary hormone produced by the adrenal medulla.

androgen: Male sex hormone, like testosterone.

cortex: The outer surface of an organ.

diuretic: Chemical that causes water to be removed from the body.

endoscope: A lighted instrument that allows doctors to see inside the body.

gland: A group of cells that release a product.

glucagon: A hormone made by islet of Langerhans cells in the pancreas that converts glycogen into glucose.

glucose: A simple sugar that is the primary energy source of cells.

glycogen: A carbohydrate that stores glucose in the muscles and liver.

gonads: Organs that produce male or female sex cells.

hormone: A chemical produced by an endocrine gland that regulates the function of a target organ.

hyper: A prefix that indicates above-normal function.

hypo: A prefix that indicates below-normal function.

insulin: A hormone made by the islet of Langerhans cells in the pancreas that helps cells take up glucose from the blood.

limbic lobe: An area of the brain that produces emotional feelings.

medulla: The inner portion of an organ.

receptor: Molecule on the surface of a cell that identifies and binds to a particular hormone.

releasing hormones: Hormones produced by the hypothalamus to regulate the pituitary gland.

secretin: A hormone produced by the small intestine that stimulates the release of digestive juices.

target organ: A group of cells that has receptors for, and is affected by, a hormone.

trophic hormone: A hormone that targets an endocrine gland.

FOR FURTHER READING

Books

Elizabeth Fong, *Body Structures and Functions.* St. Louis, MO: Times Mirror/Mosby, 1987. Provides simple and thorough description of various diseases of the human body.

David E. Larson, *Mayo Clinic Family Health Book.* New York: William Morrow, 1996. Describes in simple terms the many diseases that can affect the human body.

Susan McKeever, *The Dorling Kindersley Science Encyclopedia.* New York: Dorling Kindersley, 1994. Gives concise information on physical and biological occurrences in life. Good illustrations help to explain topics.

Mary Lou Mulvihill, *Human Diseases.* Norwalk, CT: Appleton & Lange, 1995. Provides a good description of the most common diseases of the human body.

World Book Medical Encyclopedia. Chicago: World Book, 1995. Provides a vast amount of information on the physiology of the human body systems.

Websites

About (www.about.com). Easy-to-use site that offers information on all topics, including health and medicine.

About Children's Health (www.aboutchildrenshealth.com/human body). Good information about all types of body systems.

American Diabetes Association (www.diabetes.org). Excellent resource that teaches diabetics how to cope with their disease.

CDC (www.cdc.gov/health). Information from the National Centers for Disease Control and Prevention on any topic in health.

Children's Health (www.medem.com). Information on all types of children's health issues, supplied by Medem, Inc.

Clinical Implications (www.nobel.se/medicine/laureates/1996/ illpres/implications). Contains drawings and photographs along with information on all medical topics.

Cornell Medical College (www.edcenter.med.cornell.edu). The medical college of Cornell provides a wide range of information on body systems.

Countdown for Kids Magazine (www.jdf.org/kids/cfk). Students can research any topics that interest them, including health and medicine.

Cygnus (www.cygn.com). News on technology that supports diabetics, such as the GlucoWatch Biographer.

11th Hour (www.blackwellscience.com). Valuable teacher resource for any type of information in science.

Endocrine Web.com (www.endocrineweb.com). Supplies information to help people who have diseases of the endocrine system.

Fact Monster, Learning Net Work (www.factmonstser.com). Provides information on all topics; suitable for any students. Provides good science encyclopedia.

JAMA HIV AIDS Resource Center (www.ama-assn.org). *The Journal of the American Medical Association,* published by the American Medical Association, is a great resource for any topic in medicine.

The Merck Manual Web Site (www.merck.com). This website gives a detailed explanation of body systems and diseases.

MSN Search (www.search.msn.com). Provides a science library suitable for most students.

My Thyroid.com (www.mythyroid.com). Answers questions about thyroid gland function.

Women's Health Information Center (www.ama-assn.org/special/womb/womb.htm). This site from the *Journal of the American Medical Association* covers a variety of topics related to women's health.

Yucky Kids (www.nj.com/yucky). Easy-to-read articles on a variety of science topics.

Internet Sources

American Academy of Family Physicians, "When Your Child Is Close to Puberty," 2002. www.aafp.org/afp/990700ap/990700d.html.

Jim Barlow, News Bureau, University of Illinois at Urbana-Champaign,"Growth Hormone May Boost Production of Disease-Fighting Cells in Elderly," 2002. www.news.uiuc.edu/scitips/02/0206bonecells.html.

BBC Health, "Feeling Blue," 2002. www.bbc.co.uk/health/body_chemistry/puberty_blues.shtml.

Diabetes News, "Stem Cell Research Closing in on a Diabetes Cure," 2002. www.diabetesnews.com.

Bechara Y. Ghorayeb, Otolaryngology Houston, "Minimally Invasive Radioguided Parathyroidectomy," 2002. www.ghorayeb.com/Para~ns4.html.

Health World Online, "Disorders of the Endocrine System," 2002. www.healthy.net/asp/templates/article.asp?PageType+Article&ID=673.

How Stuff Works, "How Lie Detectors Work," 2002. www.howstuffworks.com/lie-detector.htm.

Dr. Koop, "A Hassle a Day Keeps the Doctor Away," 2002. drkoop.com/template.asp?page=newsdetail&ap=93&id=505002.

Edward M. Lichten, Human Growth Hormone, Rejuvenation Medicine, "Will Growth Hormone Prove to Be the First 'Anti-Aging' Medication?" 2002. www.usdoctor.com/gh.htm.

Mayo Clinic, "Youth in a Syringe? Growth Hormone Ignites Debate," 2002. www.mayoclinic.com/findinformation/conditioncenters/invoke.cfm?objectid=671AB08.

WebMDHealth, "Stress," 2002. http://my.webmd.com/content/asset/miller_keane_31565.

WebMDHealth, "Thyroid Scan and Radioactive Iodine Uptake Test," 2002. http://my.webmd.com/encyclopedia/article/1840.52585.

WebMDHealth, "When Stress Beats Up Your Body," 2002. http://my.webmd.com/content/article/1738.51119.

INDEX

PICTURE CREDITS

ABOUT THE AUTHORS

Both Pam Walker and Elaine Wood have degrees in biology and education from colleges in Georgia. They have taught science in grades seven through twelve since the mid-1980s. Ms. Walker and Ms. Wood are coauthors of more than a dozen science-teacher resource activity books and two science textbooks.

DATE		